MW01092334

Harmonized Aromatherapy
for Seasonal Wellness

Shanti Dechen, CCAP, CAI, LMT

Founder of Aroma Apothecary Healing Arts

Academy

Shanti Dechen

The purpose of this book is to educate laypersons and health practitioners on the uses, applications, and safety of herbs, aromatherapy, and other holistic modalities.

It is sold with the understanding that neither Shanti Dechen nor Aroma Apothecary Healing Arts Academy shall have neither liability nor responsibility for any injury caused directly or indirectly by the information contained in this book. Every effort has been taken to provide accurate information. This should not be construed as medical advice. To obtain recommendations, appropriate to your particular condition, please consult a qualified health care provider.

Aroma Apothecary Healing Arts Academy

P.O. Box 690 Crestone, CO 81131

LearnAroma.com

Shanti Dechen

Acknowledgements of Gratitude

For all who have the courage to follow their own healing wisdom and to embrace it in their daily lives, with love and compassion.

This book is dedicated to my mother and father for their support to create an authentic life. With deep appreciation for introducing me to my first connection with nature, the exquisite floral radiance of my mother's flower garden, creating a deep passion for the sweet scent of herbs and flowers.

To my beautiful daughter, Jessi White; my brother and sister, Dave Anderson and Susie Christians; my nieces, Pam Neitzel and Lisa Johnston and their families. Thank you for your love, support, and teaching me unconditional love.

To all my dear friends and loved ones who have been there, supported me, and shared this beautiful journey.

To my dear Wayne Hallstrom, who makes life fun, passionate, and alive.

To all my teachers in assisting me to learn deeply about the nature of healing and that life is an amazing journey.

To all those that assisted and supported me with this book publication: editing, Haly JensenHof and Norah Charles; design, Mark Talbot; indexing, Judy Gordon. Thank you. I could not have done it without you!

To all my students of Aroma Apothecary Healing Arts Academy for sharing the passion, inspiration, and joy of aromatherapy and natural healing.

Contents

Shanti Dechen

Introduction

I was very fortunate to grow up in Colorado and to spend summers and most weekends in the Rocky Mountains. It was there that I discovered the beauty, power, and majesty of nature.

Natural healing has been a part of my daily life since I was a teenager. I started herbal investigation and attended my first holistic training at age eighteen and was hooked! Since that time, it has been a lifelong journey.

Over time, I have recognized the utmost importance of including integrative therapies and self-care maintenance into my daily life. These include aromatherapy, herbs, healthy organic nutrition, vitamin supplements, exercise, time in nature, supportive friends and family, and mental/emotion rebalancing with meditation and prayer and the use of alternative healing methods.

After decades of observing the ways of nature, it has inspired me to incorporate these insights and principles into my daily and seasonal wellness plans. I have found that working with the natural ebb and flow of nature and following the seasons has encouraged and supported vital health and balance through all of the seasons of the year. In this book, there will be an exploration of the seasonal use of herbs, essential oils, carriers, hydrosols, flower essences, holistic modalities, and a variety of aromatherapy applications that enhance optimal wellness for each season of the year.

Gaining deeper awareness into these natural cycles and the variety of plant medicine applications has assisted me to decrease stress levels, increasing my overall vitality, health, radiance, and immunity.

"Study nature, love nature, stay close to nature.
It will never fail you."
Frank Lloyd Wright

Chapter 1

Holistic and Plant Medicine

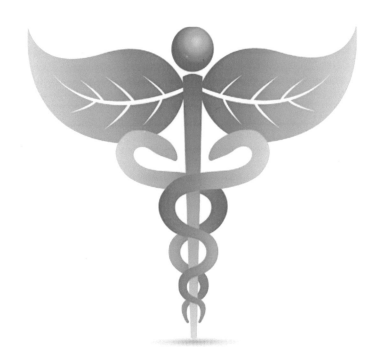

Principles of Holistic Medicine

I was first introduced to the intriguing concepts and principles of holistic medicine many decades ago. Now, years later, I have integrated many different modalities of healing together to create my template of a healing mandala that supports and nourishes my daily life. These have included a foundation of aromatherapy, herbology, meditation, nutrition, emotional rebalancing, exercise, holistic support from healing practitioners, healthy relationships with myself and others, time in nature, and the element system. Elemental patterns create foundational awareness for using holistic medicine as it relates to the patterns, characteristics, and cycles of nature.

"Holistic" comes from the Greek word 'holos' meaning whole.

A holistic approach to health works on the whole person, considering factors such as their medical history, lifestyle, nutrition, mental, emotional and spiritual states, as well as their physical body.

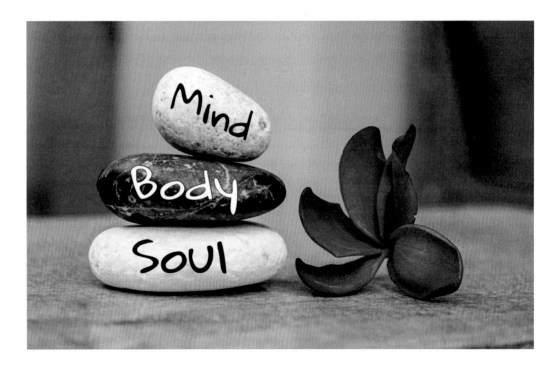

The synergy of holistic healing is expressed in different aspects of our daily lives. Below are a few aspects that I have found particularly useful in maintaining good health for my body, mind, and spirit:

- Healthy Organic Nutrition.
- Plant Medicine Allies.
- Exercise/Movement.
- Meditation and Prayer.
- Time for Self-Care.
- Time in Nature.
- Perspective of Gratitude.
- Right Livelihood.
- Enjoyment of my Work.
- Clear Communication and Harmony in my Personal and Professional Relationships.
- Team of Support: professional healers such as massage therapists, nutritionists, energy workers, chiropractors, acupuncturists, and even a holistically minded doctor/physician.

Another important aspect of holistic medicine that I have taken to heart is the belief that unconditional love and support is the most powerful healer and that the individual is ultimately responsible for his or her own health and well-being.

Other principles of holistic medicine include the following:

- Everyone has the innate power to heal.
- A patient is a person, not a disease.
- Healing takes a team approach involving the patient and doctor and addresses all aspects of a person's life using a variety of healthcare practices.
- Treatment consists of rebalancing the cause of the condition, not just alleviating the symptoms.
- Holistic practitioners use a variety of treatment techniques to help their patients take responsibility for their well-being and achieve optimal health.

Holistic medicine practitioners believe that the whole person is made of a sum of interdependent parts and if one aspect is not working correctly, then all of the other parts will be affected. In this way, if people have imbalances (physical, emotional, or spiritual) in their lives, they can negatively impact their overall health.

A holistic doctor or practitioner may use all forms of health care, from conventional medication to alternative therapies, to rebalance, not fix, a patient.

For example, when a person who is suffering from migraine headaches pays a visit to a holistic doctor, instead of walking out solely with medications, the doctor will likely take a look at all the potential factors. These factors may include other health problems, nutritional habits, sleep habits, stress levels, personal issues, and preferred spiritual practices.

The treatment plan may involve drugs to relieve symptoms but also lifestyle modifications to help prevent the headaches from recurring.

Depending on the practitioner's training, these may include:

- Patient education, including lifestyle changes and self-care to promote daily wellness.
- Nutrition.
- Exercise/movement therapies.
- Counseling or psychotherapy.
- Relationship or spiritual counseling.

Complementary and alternative therapies can also include: aromatherapy, herbology, acupressure, acupuncture, chiropractic, naturopathy, homeopathy, massage therapy, reflexology, yoga, tai chi, qigong, and energy medicine, to name a few modalities.

The habits and patterns that make up our daily lives are very influential in our resulting overall health. It is useful to begin by observing our regular habit patterning.

It is easier to assess our lives and make changes if we begin with one step at a time. This might entail increasing your daily water intake or exercise. Once you establish a new habit pattern for yourself then you can add another beneficial change. If we try to make too many changes at once, there may be an internal conflict that sabotages any change taking place.

Is there one thing you would like to change that would be beneficial for your overall health?

One easy way to establish a new healthy pattern is to combine it with one of your favorite essential oils. As we know, aromatherapy has a unique ability to connect with the limbic system in the brain within twenty seconds of inhalation. Olfaction is the process of the brain perceiving odor. The limbic system is where our memories, instincts, and vital functions are controlled and processed.

A simple technique of re-anchoring is to inhale the beautiful scent of an essential oil every time you do something beneficial and positive for yourself. This inhalation technique can become a powerful support to encourage new healthy habits.

Connection with Your Own Healing Nature

Plants are deeply connected with our existence on earth. They can heal us, protect us, and be our food and medicine. They inform us of both the harmony and imbalances within ourselves, and they can open us up to the microcosmic expansion, which expresses the essential features, in miniature, of the characteristic qualities or features of something much more significant.

There are many effective ways to connect with nature. It starts with deepening a connection with ourselves.

Every plant, seed, tree, flower, and bush has their unique qualities, not only the typical uses or chemistry, but they also contain a deeper level of sensory awareness. When we can find a particular attraction or connection that guides us to our plant allies, we feel nurtured and soothed in our physical, mental, emotional and spiritual selves.

I have always felt it is essential, as an aromatherapist and natural health practitioner, to build relationships with the herbs and essential oils that I work with in creating aromatherapy and herbal formulations. Over many decades this intention has inspired me to be more in tune with the innate knowledge of plants and myself.

It was in my childhood that I began to nurture a connection with nature and plants. Some of my first memories are the beauty and wonder of my mother's beautiful rose garden, the intoxicating scent of the lily of the valley in our yard, the conifer trees in the mountains of Colorado, and the orange tree flowers in bloom during our family vacations in California. These flowers, from the bitter orange tree, are neroli (*Citrus aurantium var. amara*), an essential oil of exquisite radiance.

Still today, the conifer trees create a sense of grounding and comfort for me, especially the wafting scent of the trees in the forest after a rain shower. When I sit and connect with the pinion pine (*Pinus edulis*) trees that are vast in my backyard, I reflect on the form of the tree, the aromatic scent, the needles, and branches.

The branches of the conifer trees remind me of the structure that is similar to the human respiratory system, and the shape of the branches and needles are like a scrub brush. In harmony with its structure, these tree essential oils are useful for clearing congestion in the respiratory, circulatory, lymphatic, and emotional systems.

On the herbal website SusunWeed.com, I recently read a blog article by Jane Sherry in which she describes all the ways in which we have incorporated nature into our everyday language.

- "We say we have put down roots when we have established ourselves and feel at home in our surroundings.
- When we move to a new land or a new job, we say we have found new soil in which to grow; we are transplants.
- We say that we are planting seeds for the future when we are germinating new ideas, cultivating new friends and relationships.
- We say we are branching out when we try something new.
- When we make big changes in our lives, we have breakthroughs. We say that we are breaking new ground.
- As we incorporate these new ways into our lives our habits change and we say we are growing new roots."[1]

How true this is, that we connect our thoughts and experiences of our daily lives with the language of plants and nature. Without a doubt, plants impact the way we think about ourselves and the world around us.

Creating Your Plant Allies

When we are grounded and centered, we feel a deeper connection to others, our environment, and ourselves. As you connect with different plants and trees, it encourages an activation of your senses, enhancing the intuitive mind rather than rational thinking.

For myself, one of my favorite colors is blue, so naturally, I am attracted to blue flowers like borage (*Borago officinalis*) and also "blue" essential oils like yarrow (*Acheilia millefolium*) and German chamomile (*Matricaria recutita*). All of these plants have the medicinal qualities of anti-inflammatories, which is also the nature of blue, cool, and calming water.

What plant or essential oil assists you to feel grounded and centered?

If you don't have a garden you can start with an aromatic houseplant like rosemary (*Rosmarinus officinalis*), basil (*Ocimum basilicum*), lavender (*Lavandula officinalis*) or rose geranium (*Pelargonium var. roseum*). You can begin to notice the color, size, and texture of a leaf, stem, and flower.

If this plant is aromatic, rub your fingers on a leaf and smell the fragrant scent. Is it sharp, soft, invigorating, calming? What is your impression, and does it remind you of another time in your life?

As you take care of this plant you will notice what kind of soil and nutrients it likes, the amount of sunlight, and how much water it needs. This type of awareness on the outside can also assist us to deepen the inner healing wisdom of our own needs.

Another way to make a stronger connection with nature is to notice more closely the change of the seasons, and what happens to the cycle of plants. This awareness can provide a more natural rhythm in our own lives. These plant cycles are reflected in human beings in a longer time span of birth, adolescence, maturity, and old age.

You can begin by noticing a difference in your activity in each season; summer is a higher time of activity whereas the winter is generally a time for self-reflection and nurturing, restoration of our physical and emotional being.

As you reflect on creating a profound connection with nature, whether it is a plant, herb, or essential oil, may you find harmony, balance, and healing.

Plant Relationships

Humanity has had a symbiotic relationship with plants and herbs since the beginning of time. Healing with medicinal plants is as old as humankind itself. The ancients understood what was happening inside the body by comparing it to what was happening outside in nature and related these natural laws of nature to every level and situation of phenomena.

They saw the microcosm (small universe) as a mirror image of the macrocosm (big universe). This underlying philosophy recognized the interconnectedness between humans, nature, and the world, and understood the vital importance of maintaining balance and harmony between human beings and their environment.

The wonders of natural plant medicine are here to assist us in maintaining health and vibrancy.

Since ancient times, herbal medicine has been used by many different cultures throughout the world to treat dis-ease and to assist bodily functions. An "herb" is any plant or plant part used for its medicinal, therapeutic value. Herbal medicine, also called herbology, herbalism, botanical medicine, or phytomedicine, refers to utilizing a plant's seeds, roots, leaves, flowers, berries, or bark for medicinal healing purposes.

Medicinal plants, which humans have used throughout history to assist or lessen symptoms from an illness, have similar chemical properties as conventional pharmaceutical drugs. We have evolved for thousands of years using plants; and our bodies are better suited to digest, absorb, and metabolize these plant-based foods and medicines.

The plant kingdom is genuinely full of wondrous treasures and fantastic healing medicinals.

Most of us think of plants as being silent and simplistic. They make food from sunshine, photosensitize, and in turn feed animals and humans. However, plants are very complex and are not as sedentary or solitary as we imagine. Even though they do not have eyes or ears, they do have unique ways of perceiving their environment and adapting accordingly. Plants actively respond to the elements, nutrients, herbivores grazing on flora, and other predators around them through extensive and sophisticated communication and cooperation.

Plant Intelligence

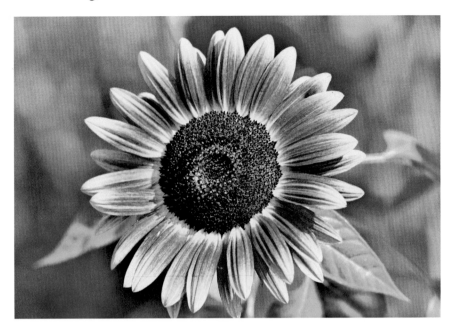

Could plants have a memory or a nervous system?

In the BBC documentary, "How Plants Communicate & Think," Francis Halle, a renowned botanist and emeritus professor at the University of Montpellier states, "The more genes an organism has, the more evolved we perceive that it is."[2]

However, to the surprise of many botanists, plants have more genes to adapt than humans. Plants and animals have evolved together and have a symbiotic relationship.

Bees, birds, insects, worms, ants, and nutrients feed the plants, the plants feed the animals, and the animals assist in carrying the plant spores, pollinating the plants and dispersing their seed. The plants' rules of survival have developed through adaptation, communication, and cooperation.

Botanist Dieter Volkmann, Ph.D. is a leader in the research of plant intelligence at the University of Bonn, Germany. He is studying the way plants perceive and react to their environment; the ways they find light, air, and nutrients; as well as how they communicate with each other. Not only are these perceptions and reactions observed as sensations by plants, but there is also consciousness in the plant world.

Plant Memory

Do plants have a type of central nervous system that responds to stimulation, perception, and previous experience?

This next section may seem a bit technical, but it is important to convey the interconnectedness of plants to other plants, plants to animals, and plants to humans.

Recent advances in plant cell biology and neuroscience reveal surprising similarities between plant cells and neurons. "They have signal input and signal output poles, secrete signaling molecules via robust endocytosis-driven vesicle recycling apparatus, and are capable of sensory perception and integration of these multiple sensory perceptions into adaptive actions that serve for the survival of organisms, harboring these cells specialized for signaling and communication. Moreover, neurons and plant cells have in common abilities to generate spontaneously action potentials, which convey electric signaling across tissues of multicellular organisms."[3]

In other words, plants can remember reactions, store a specific chemical signal, and respond at a later time. Dr. František Baluška is a biologist who has been studying the brain theory of plant roots. Dr. Baluška has found a physiological function at the tip of the plant root that can integrate chemical sensitivities for adaptation. There is also a transition zone in the upper area of a plant root that contains cells that are also found in animal muscle tissue. In animals, these cells interact with the synapses of nerves, as well as with memory and thought.

The roots of a plant can process complex information, much like our nervous system, to communicate with the rest of the plant stimulating it to flourish or to go dormant. The plant's neurobiology is similar in structure and molecular level to a vertebrate's neuronal system. Plant cells may be different in function but are very similar to neurons and synapses that form nerve circuits in animals. The structures may be different in plants, animals, and humans, but the results are almost identical in helping each life form function and thrive.

Plant Defense

Over 400,000 species of plants cover the earth. Each one is remarkable, but none can survive on the planet alone. All life depends on connections or interdependencies that are vital for unique eco-systems to survive. Trees and plants react to nutrients that are transported by fluids in the air and the soil. Also, by communicating through fungi and algae networks, plants extend their roots to gather nutrients and alert other plants in the area of any damage or infections.

"Mycorrhizal describes the mutually beneficial relationship between the plant and root fungus. These specialized fungi colonize plant roots and extend far into the soil. Mycorrhizal fungal filaments in the soil are truly extensions of root systems and are more effective in nutrient and water absorption than the roots themselves. More than 90 percent of plant species in natural areas form a symbiotic relationship with the beneficial mycorrhizal fungi.

This plant/fungi relationship increases the surface absorption area of roots from 100 to 1,000 times, thereby significantly improving the ability of the plant to access soil resources. Several miles of fungal filaments can be present in less than a thimbleful of soil. Mycorrhizal fungi increase nutrient uptake not only by increasing the surface absorbing area of the roots but also by releasing powerful enzymes into the earth that dissolve hard-to-capture nutrients; such as organic nitrogen, phosphorus, iron and other "tightly bound" soil nutrients.

This extraction process is particularly important in plant nutrition and explains why non-mycorrhizal plants require high levels of fertilization to maintain their health. Mycorrhizal fungi form an intricate web that captures and assimilates nutrients, conserving the nutrient capital in soils."[4]

In the growth process, plants produce a variety of compounds that can be divided into primary metabolites and secondary metabolites. Primary metabolites are essential for the survival of the plant and include sugars, proteins, and amino acids. Plants have their own survival mechanisms and the ability to create their own antibodies.

Secondary metabolites were once believed to be waste products. They are not essential to the plant's survival, but the plant does suffer without them. For plants to stay healthy, secondary metabolism plays a crucial role in keeping all of the plant's systems working correctly.

A typical role of secondary metabolites in plants is as a defense mechanism. Secondary metabolites also act as signals for symbiotic bacteria; attractants for pollinators and seed-dispersing animals; allopathic agents in natural habitats; physical and chemical barriers to abiotic stressors, such as UV and evaporation; and endogenous regulators of plant growth hormones. Many secondary metabolites are also useful for healing in humans, such as essential oils.

Plants have their own unique language, at a molecular level, to communicate with each other, which helps plants to prevent disease and repel pests.

Humans are very much like plants; they draw in needed energy to nourish physical, emotional and spiritual states. How can we connect this natural healing potential to ourselves?

Dr. Olivia Bader-Lee suggests that the field of bioenergetics is ever evolving and that studies on the plant and animal world will soon translate and demonstrate what energy metaphysicians have known all along: "That humans can heal each other simply through energy transfer, just as plants do. Humans can absorb and heal through other humans, animals, and any part of nature. That's why being around nature is often uplifting, energizing, and healing for so many people.

When energy studies become more advanced in the coming years, we will eventually see this translated to human beings as well," states Bader-Lee. "The human organism is very much like a plant, it draws needed energy to feed emotional states, and this can essentially energize cells or cause increases in cortisol and catabolize cells depending on the emotional trigger."[5]

"Plants have scientifically been shown to draw alternative sources of energy from other plants. Plants influence each other in many ways, and they communicate through 'nanomechanical oscillations,' vibrations on the tiniest atomic or molecular scale."[6]   This is as close as you can get to telepathic communication!

Learning from the essential nature of the marvelous plant kingdom to adapt, communicate, and cooperate within our own relationships, generates an inter-dependent partnership with plants in which we can balance and heal ourselves.

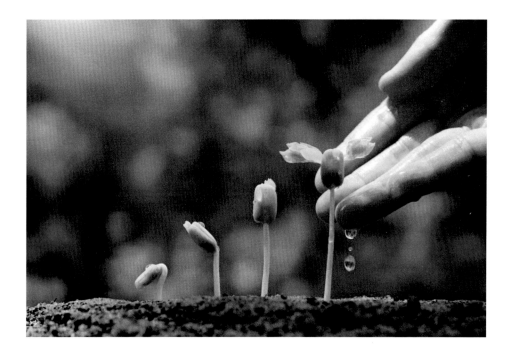

Chapter 2

Integrated Self-Care

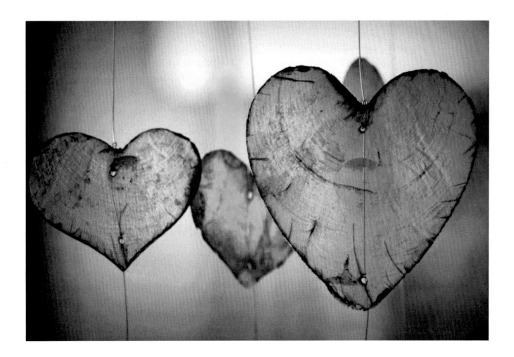

Empowered Self-Care

Self-care is crucial to our physical, mental, emotional, and spiritual well-being. It encompasses a wide variety of ways that we can empower ourselves to enhance our daily well-being and cope effectively with stress.

As the ancient Greek philosopher Socrates mentioned, "Wisdom begins with wonder." To know yourself is the first step to gaining healing wisdom. Plato also alluded to the fact that understanding 'thyself,' would yield a more significant outcome in understanding the true nature of human life.

Knowing yourself is not a destination but a path to self-discovery and awareness.

To some, this may seem indulgent, especially for women, because we are generally raised to care about others more than ourselves. It has taken me many years, and close to adrenal exhaustion, to recognize that before I can take care of and love others, I need to begin by doing this for myself.

One of the first things to consider is to maintain and support a healthy relationship with yourself. I finally recognized that I am ultimately my best support and cheerleader in this game called life. Over time I have identified different aspects of self-care. The very basics that I include in my daily life are: drinking plenty of water, healthy nutrition, exercise, taking time for myself in nature and relaxing, deepening close relationships, and getting enough sleep.

It is useful to lay the groundwork and habitual patterning on a daily basis when we feel our best. Then, when we feel stressed or imbalanced, we can fall back on these healthy habits.

**" When we are unable to find tranquility within ourselves,
it is useless to seek it elsewhere."
La Rochefoucauld**

Creating balance in our daily lives is a step-by-step journey. There are many ways to explore and integrate self-care and learn to be your own health and wellness coach.

Here are some basics of encouraging self-care:

- **Knowing your self-worth** helps to boosts your confidence and self-esteem. A useful saying or affirmation I learned from my teacher, Lar Short, was a way to connect with myself in the morning. As you look in the mirror you can say to yourself, or out loud, "I look good, I sound great, I feel myself radiate." Become your own best friend.

- **Let go of overworking**. Balance work and home life. It took time for me to learn that it is NOT a virtue to work all the time. Overworking was stressful and exhausting. I became less productive, disorganized, and emotionally depleted. I also recognized that overdoing, or continual multi-tasking for long periods of time, can lead to many health problems, from anxiety and depression, to insomnia, adrenal stress, and heart diseases.

- **Set the basis of healthy self-care habits**, like taking breaks, going into nature, and taking time for yourself. By establishing personal and professional boundaries, you will you stay aware, inspired and healthy.

Here are some key components I have anchored into my daily life that are supportive and nourishing.

- Self-care.
- Herbs: teas, capsules, tinctures, & infusions.
- Healthy nutrition: food is your daily medicine.
- Aromatherapy.
- Vitamin supplements.
- Exercise.
- Holistic treatment modalities.
- Time in nature.
- Supportive friends and family.
- Mental and emotional balancing.
- Positive thoughts about self.
- Spiritual alignment- meditation & prayer.

As a board-certified massage therapist, I have studied numerous types of bodywork and holistic healing methods. On a regular basis I also receive various types of healing work as an integral part of my wellness foundation. These treatments assist me to relax deeply and to obtain feedback on different issues or imbalances within my bodymind. They reduce overall aches, pains, and stagnate energies that can be quickly relieved before there is a chronic problem or imbalance.

"Our bodies are our gardens to which our wills are gardeners."
William Shakespeare

Variations of Massage and Bodywork

Below is a brief description of the most common types of massage and other holistic healing modalities.

Swedish Massage- the most common type of massage offered in gyms, spas, and some wellness centers. Swedish massage is focused on the Western concepts of anatomy and physiology, compared to the energy-centered style more common in Asian forms of massage.

Deep Tissue Bodywork- a slower, deeper type of therapeutic massage that focuses on releasing adhesions in the deeper layers of muscle and connective tissue.

Deep tissue bodywork can also include these other modalities:

Neuromuscular (the junction of nerves and muscles): a type of bodywork that uses trigger points to release muscular pain symptoms.

Myofascial Release- (originated by John F. Barnes, PT. LMT.) a safe and effective bodywork technique that involves applying gentle, sustained pressure into myofascial connective tissue restrictions to eliminate pain and restore motion.

Sports Massage- geared towards athletes. Focused on areas of the body that are overused and stressed from repetitive, and often aggressive, movements.

Rolfing and Structural Integration- similar types of bodywork that focus on correcting postural and structural deviations by working on fascia (connective tissue surrounding muscles, groups of muscles, blood vessels, organs, and nerves). Fascia is designed to be elastic and free-moving with muscles and bones. If there is an obstruction due to injury, stress, or repetitive motion, the tightened fascia pulls the muscles and skeleton out of proper alignment, which can cause pain, discomfort, fatigue, and postural alignment.

Hot Stone- a stand-alone therapy or combined with other forms of massage. The heated basalt stones used in this modality are very relaxing and can quickly loosen tight muscles so that the therapist can release deeper areas of muscle tension more effectively.

Lymphatic Drainage- a system using very light pressure and long, gentle, rhythmic strokes to increase the flow of lymph and reduce toxins in the body. The lymphatic system is part of your body's immune system and helps fight infection.

Chi Nei Tsang Abdominal Therapy- the abdomen is the main center of our digestion, circulation, elimination, and lymphatic systems. Chi Nei Tsang is an abdominal massage used to correct imbalances of the muscles and connective tissue in the internal organs. There are specific techniques to clear tension and obstructions from each of the internal organs.

Benefits of Chi Nei Tsang include:

- Improved digestion and assimilation.
- Improved elimination.
- Detoxification and strengthening of weak or stressed organs.
- Boosting of the immune system.
- Increased ease and fullness of breathing.
- Release of physical and emotional blockages.

Mayan Abdominal Therapy- an external, non-invasive, and nurturing treatment of the abdomen and pelvic area that gently guides internal organs into their appropriate anatomical positions for optimum health and well-being.

Abdominal therapies are *not* recommended during pregnancy or for those with pacemakers.

Clothed bodywork

Thai Massage- an ancient healing system that combines acupressure, rhythmic compression of the muscle tissues, and assisted yoga postures.

Shiatsu- a therapy of Japanese origin based on the same principles as acupuncture. Techniques include kneading, pressing, smoothing, tapping, and various stretching methods. The focus of shiatsu stimulates acupressure points on the body to improve the flow of energy and help regain balance. Shiatsu is usually a clothed therapy done on a mat placed on the floor or a low massage table.

Reflexology- sessions generally focus on applied pressure points on the feet, hands, and ears. Since the body is a hologram of nature, the whole is reflected in each part. Every microsystem found in different parts of the body contains information needed to treat the whole body. This information is stored everywhere in the body and is accessed through known reflexes in the face, eyes (iridology), ears (auricular), teeth, spine (associated points), navel, abdomen, the limbs, hands, and feet.

Craniosacral Therapy - developed in the 1970's by John Upledger M.D., a doctor of osteopathy, as a form of cranial osteopathy. This technique uses gentle touch to palpate the joints of the cranium. A practitioner of cranial-sacral therapy may also apply light touches to a patient's spine and pelvic bones. It is useful to reduce migraines, headaches, chronic neck, shoulder and back pain, motor-coordination impairments, brain, and spinal injuries.

Acupuncture and Acupressure- in Chinese medicine there are over 365 points on the human body that are connected by fourteen central pathways called meridians. These meridians conduct energy, or qi (pronounced "chi"), between the surface of the body and the internal organs and they are connected with each other, ensuring the free-flow of qi throughout the whole body.

If a problem arises in any of the meridians, imbalance affects the flow of qi. Acupuncture and acupressure modalities are used to restore balance so that the qi can flow with regularity and the body's energy can resume its normal function. Even though the meridians are located externally on the body, the qi turns inward, nourishing the internal organs. Stimulation by thin needles in acupuncture, or by finger or thumb pressure of acupressure points, can rebalance and correct the qi pathways, stimulating physiological change across the body.

Emotional Freedom Technique (EFT),- also known as "Tapping" is a self-applied emotional release acupressure technique that quickly and gently releases negative emotions and beliefs. EFT utilizes meridian points that are stimulated by tapping on them with the fingertips, addressing the body's energy and healing power.

Energy Work- subtle types of healing that, for the most part, involve a light touch or hands being held above the client's body. Below is a brief description of the most common types of energy work.

Resonance Alchemy- a powerful resonance frequency healing technique, developed by Katherine Parker. This unique holistic energy medicine system uses the frequencies of universal sacred syllables to create a higher vibrational field. The results can reduce stress, develop greater energetic coherence, clear energy blockages, facilitate physical, emotional and spiritual healing.

Pranic Healing- an energy healing system based on the fundamental principle that the body has the innate ability to heal itself. Pranic Healing utilizes "life force," "energy," or "prana" to accelerate the body's inborn ability to correct its own imbalances.

Reiki- a light touch or off-the-body therapy that moves the energy flow through affected parts of the energy field and charges them with positive energy.

Medical Qigong- used either as a primary therapy or as an adjunct therapy with acupuncture, acupressure, and massage. A medical qigong therapist may recommend qigong exercises using physical movement, breathing methods, and mental intention to correct and restore the function in the body.

Mind and Emotions

**"The natural state of our body is relaxed and free of pain.
The mind is at peace emanating spacious inspiration and pure joy."
Shanti Dechen**

Psychoneuroimmunology (PNI) is the study of the effect of the mind on health and resistance to disease. **Psycho** relates to the mind and emotions, **neuro** relates to the nervous system, and **immunology** relates to the immune system.

PNI researchers have studied how emotions and thoughts impact the brain, hormones, nervous system, and the immune system's ability to protect. Research has shown that people in stressful situations have measurable changes in physical responses to injury, whether it be slow wound healing, a higher incidence of infection, or a worse prognosis as in a debilitating illness. These are promising scientific discoveries on the mind-body connection.

Many things happen in our lives to disrupt our emotional balance and create thoughts and feelings of stress, anxiety, or sadness. Unresolved negative thoughts can remain in the body and affect every area of our lives, from sleepless nights to poor health, and on to relationship or financial challenges. Emotional stress is linked to chronic inflammation, lowered immune function, increased blood pressure, and altered brain chemistry.

Being aware of our thoughts, feelings, and behaviors is the first step toward maintaining emotional health. People who are emotionally healthy have learned ways to cope with stress brought on by challenges that are part of life.

A healthy routine of adequate rest, proper nutrition, exercise, and letting go of adverse situations can be enhanced by the use of herbs, aromatherapy and integrative medicine.

Healing Deeper Emotions

There are times when emotional pain can be severe, inhibiting our ability to enjoy life. A divorce, the death of a loved one, physical abuse, or caring for someone very ill can trigger emotional reactions and create significant problems in the form of physical pain or disease. To heal these distressing emotions, one needs to access them in his or her conscious awareness where they can ultimately be released.

What can we do about troubling or negative emotions?

I have used meditation techniques for over forty years to deepen my connection with the spaciousness and healing aspects of my mind, assisting me to view my thoughts and feelings with an unbiased attitude. When my overall attitude changes, then the whole atmosphere of my mind changes, even the very nature of my thoughts and emotions. Meditation also influences my body wellness, clearing congestion and stagnation that can create illness and other physical issues.

There are many powerful and effective ways of working with emotional pain so that it can be cleared from your body, mind, and spirit. A simple way to start is through a practice of gratitude.

Choosing Gratitude

When I wake up in the morning, I take a moment to check in and see how my bodymind feels. If I am stiff then I take a few minutes to breathe deeply, stretch my body and awaken the connection between my body, mind, emotions, and spirit. I set an intention for my day, which also helps to lay a clear path. An intention is a guiding principle for how I want to be, live, and express myself in the world, throughout my day, or in any area of my life.

I usually start my daily intentions with a sense of appreciation and gratitude for the simple things in my life:

- Clean water.
- Nourishing food: choose organic, non-GMO.
- Beautiful home.
- Loving friends and family.
- Successful business.

Some useful intentions to start with:

- Thank you for the guidance to be present and loving in this day.
- Thank you for the confidence to be me.
- Surround me with caring and compassionate people.
- May all my connections be meaningful.
- Open my heart and mind to give and receive love freely.

For years I have cultivated the daily approach of gratitude for my life and have witnessed the increased blossoming of compassion, love, and success throughout each day. The intention process assists me to make clear choices and to attract more goodness.

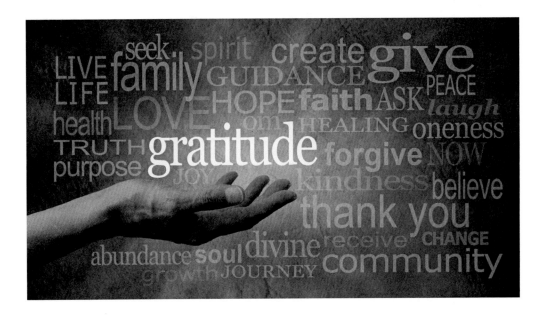

"Intention is the starting point of every dream. It is the creative power that fulfills all of our needs, whether for money, relationships, spiritual awakening, or love."
Deepak Chopra

Mindfulness Moment

Training your bodymind awareness on a daily basis will assist in developing healthy patterns, strengthening your immune system, enhancing overall radiance, and experiencing the vitality of life.

To bring yourself into a receptive state of mind, find a quiet space. You can be seated or lying down, but it will help if your spine is straight.

- Choose your favorite relaxing essential oil and put a couple of drops on a cotton pad or in a nasal inhaler. Breathe deeply, allowing the essence to penetrate. Deepen the breath to penetrate into your lungs, expanding your abdomen and back ribs.

- Close your eyes and bring your gaze to focus on your navel and feel the centering power of this gesture.

- Next, bring your attention to the bottoms of your feet and feel the connection to the earth.

- Continue to focus your awareness on your breath into the upper chest, abdomen and back relaxing and letting go of the tension.

- As you feel a sense of grounding and are more relaxed, slowly open your eyes and move forward in a relaxed manner.

Fostering a sense of gratitude for what we have makes us better able to cope with stress, have more positive emotions, and allows for a more joyful life.

"Watch your thoughts; they become words.
Watch your words; they become actions.
Watch your actions; they become habits.
Watch your habits; they become character.
Watch your character; it becomes your destiny."
Lao Tzu

Creating Clear Boundaries

Becoming grounded in your body is essential to creating clear boundaries, especially when you are a sensitive type, like myself. Throughout the years I've had people say, "Oh, you're too sensitive," which turned out to be a blessing in disguise. In my forty years as a holistic health practitioner, my sensitivities became an empathic skill. It has been enriching working with others and being able to read their bodies and to have clarity about what was going on in their minds and emotions. Over time, with these sensitivities, I have also learned that it is vital to have clear boundaries.

- Personal boundaries reflect self-love and self-esteem.
- Be yourself with integrity and take responsibility for yourself.
- In communication, be truthful and say what you mean. Even in a challenging situation you can learn to communicate honestly with grace and compassion.
- Know the core values that define you. What is important to you?
- Be respectful, kind, and compassionate toward yourself and others.
- Be truthful.
- If we are not attached to the outcome we can change our responses to situations.
- Honor your needs and limits.
- It is ok to say, "NO."
- You cannot change others, but you can improve yourself and your reactions.

You are in charge of your moment-to-moment choices.
Empower yourself!

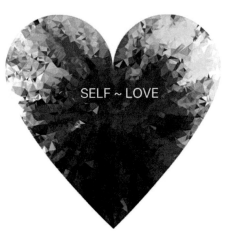

SELF ~ LOVE

Chapter 3

USING
MEDICINAL PLANTS

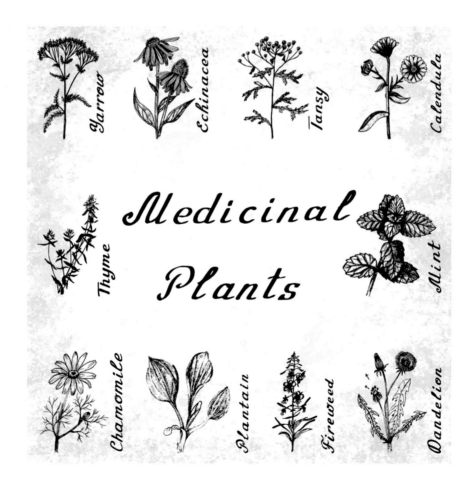

Historical Use of Medicinal Plants

Herbs, flower essences, hydrosols, essential oils, and holistic treatments encourage an environment for healing. These allies provide support in integrating and releasing pent-up feelings and tensions. We must free these trapped energies before we can genuinely receive positive feelings, love, and healing. While these remedies will not do all the inner work for us, meditation, journaling, counseling, and being present with yourself can significantly facilitate the process towards a genuinely healthy and radiant state of being.

Since ancient times, herbal medicine has been used throughout the world and by many cultures to treat illnesses and to assist bodily functions. The connection between humans and their search for botanical medicine dates from the distant past. There is a vast amount of evidence, from various sources pointing to this relationship: written documents, preserved monuments, and even original plant medicines.

Indigenous cultures, such as African and American Indian, have always used herbs in their healing rituals. Other cultures developed traditional medical systems, such as Ayurveda from India and traditional Chinese medicine, in which herbal therapies were integrated.

We have evolved for thousands of years by using plants, and our bodies are better suited to digesting, absorbing, and metabolizing these plant-based foods and medicines.

This natural healing method of herbology is based on the systematic use of plants or plant extracts that are ingested as tea, capsules, tinctures, and flower essences, or used for topical application in compresses and infusions.

Why Use Herbs?

Herbal medicine's effectiveness and safety has stood the test of time. For thousands of years, humans have learned to pursue remedies in seeds, roots, leaves, fruits, berries, flowers, bark, and other parts of the plants for their healing. The popularity and longevity of herbal use throughout the world is undeniable evidence of the healing power of plants against dis-ease and illnesses.

Herbology is only part of a complete holistic perspective on health, which goes beyond the standard western medical view of cause and effect. This comprehensive perspective also takes into consideration factors of your daily life, including environment, healthy organic nutrition, lifestyle (sedentary or active), daily stressors, habitual patterning of physical, mental and emotional attitudes, and spiritual perspective.

Developing a healthy attitude is a large part of the process in seeing your life and problems from a holistic perspective. Dis-ease that is healed naturally leaves a person stronger and better able to adapt to situations in the future.

As mentioned by Lao Tzu, in the *Tao Te Ching,* there are three great treasures to cultivate for personal health and wellness:

> **"Simplicity, patience, and compassion.**
> **These three are your greatest treasures.**
> **Simplicity in actions and thoughts, you return to the source of being.**
> **Patience with both friends and enemies,**
> **you accord with the way things are.**
> **Compassion toward yourself, you reconcile all beings in the world."**
> **Lao Tzu**

It is imperative to recognize the natural symbiotic relationship that we have with plants, and their healing nature, to restore balance beyond a cause and effect perspective. Herbal remedies assist the body to stimulate, regulate, adapt, and promote self-healing as nature intended. Both traditional and modern researchers believe that herbs, when used correctly, encourage the body to heal itself.

For an herbal remedy to be entirely successful it has to include recognition and communication with the inner self. The full embodiment of healing always integrates the body, mind, emotions, and spirit.

One of the most important things to keep at the forefront of your mind when working with plants, in any capacity, is that they *are* intelligent beings. They can feel and respond to your energy and intention. If you have a plant that you love, that plant will do very well, even in conditions that are less than ideal. Plants will let you know what they need, but it is our job to listen to what they are telling us.

Take a moment to visualize your favorite plant or flower. What emotions or feelings does this image evoke for you? Do you feel joy? Energized? Comforted?

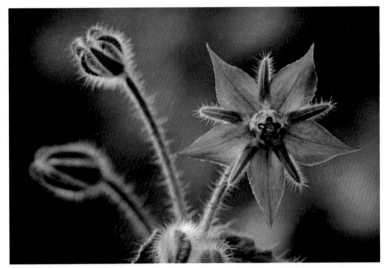

This last summer, Borage (*Borago officinalis*) became one of my favorite plants growing in my botanical garden. The first thing that attracted me was the beautiful star-shaped flowers. Looking at the flowers resonated with my heart center, and I felt very joyful and relaxed every time I was collecting the beautiful flowers. I used the fresh flowers to add to my salads and then to dry and infuse into jojoba oil for my aromatherapy facial serums.

The stems of borage feel a bit rough, which tells me it could be used in reducing inflammation and to ease those rough spots within the body and mind.

I am also aware that borage seeds contain an abundant level of gamma-linolenic acid or GLA, an essential fatty acid, which has proven benefits in reducing inflammation.

Borage oil is an excellent choice to add into face serum blends because of its restorative power for prematurely aged skin, psoriasis, and eczema. It reduces damage and inflammation from ultraviolet rays. Menstrual complaints, PMS, menopausal discomfort, inflammatory conditions, and heart imbalances also seem to benefit from the use of borage oil.

Connecting with the borage plant is a simple example of the emotional intelligence of an herb. Each herb has its personality, medicinal qualities, and energetic medicine for healing our physical and emotional bodies.

There are a fantastic variety of applications to utilize herbal medicines. Gathering knowledge from the study and experience of herbs is *essential* to choosing the correct use of botanical medicine for each person and situation.

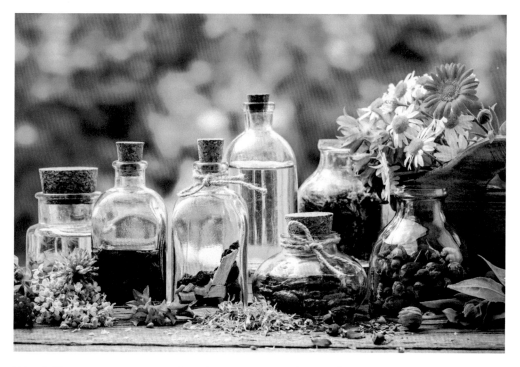

The following pages are a brief overview of the methods of utilizing medicinal plants. The following seasonal chapters will explore these methods in more detail. The choice of plant remedies selected for the season is a personal and subjective interpretation; each herb has different qualities in its variations of use. These suggestions may vary from herbal remedies that are associated with other elements and seasons from different traditions. I encourage you to take what you learn here and expand your knowledge of medicinal plants in whichever direction your inquisitiveness leads you.

Uses of Herbs

The applications of herbs can include: fresh, dried, capsules, tinctures, infused, flower essences, distilled into hydrosols, and essential oils.

Herbs- Used fresh or dried in cooking as spices, teas, and herbal medicines.

Herbal Preparations

Herbal Infusion: Pour one quart of boiling water over two tablespoons of herb(s) and let it steep for twenty minutes. Keep the lid on tightly. Drink three to four cups daily, or as needed.

Root Infusion: Use one to two tablespoons of a chosen root per quart of water. Pour boiling water over the root and let the infusion sit for thirty minutes, or even overnight. Keep the pot well covered. Strain and drink four cups daily.

Herbal Decoction: A decoction is a method of extraction for stems, roots, and bark in boiling water to dissolve the chemicals of the material. Add one tablespoon of dried herbs or two tablespoons of fresh herbs to one cup of boiling water. Reduce heat to simmer for 20-30 minutes. Strain off the herbs. Drink 1/4 -1/2 cup as needed, adding additional hot water and a sweetener, like honey or stevia, if it has a pungent taste.

If you are combining both herbs and roots, decoct the roots first, and then turn off the heat. Then, add the leaves and flowers, cover tightly, and infuse as long as desired. Strain and drink four cups daily.

Vegetable Capsules- Used for dried herbs when a stronger internal remedy or duration is needed, or if herbs taste particularly unpleasant.

Tinctures or Extracts- Tinctures, also known as herbal extracts, are produced from both aromatic and non-aromatic plants. Tinctures are a stronger herbal application that is quickly absorbed into the digestive system. Tinctures include herbs that have been extracted into a base of alcohol, vegetable glycerin, or apple cider vinegar. They are taken internally and can be added to tea, juice, water, or into smoothies.

Infusion- Infusion or maceration is another method of extraction that is used for plants that cannot be steam distilled or extracted through pressing, such as seeds and nuts. This process is utilized when the plant matter is non-aromatic or would be too expensive for the amount of oil produced by distillation.

To create an infusion, the flower heads or plant matter is collected, dried, and then covered in a vegetable-based oil of either jojoba (*Simmondsia chinensis*) or olive (*Olea europaea*) oil. I prefer to use these particular carrier oils, which have a long shelf life over other carrier oils. There are also plant infusions done in an alcohol or vegetable glycerin base.

Flower Essences- A water-based infusion of fresh flowers. Used to balance emotions and calm mental states. Flower essences can be taken for short-term benefits: to increase clarity, calming, and confidence. Or, they can be taken long-term, over a regular, consistent basis to accelerate personal growth and enhance awareness. If you still have fresh flowers in your garden, processing them into flower essences can be a fantastic way to soothe the emotions and instill a healthy balance throughout the year.

A useful reference book on this herbal remedy is *Flower Essence Reparatory* by Patricia A. Kaminski and Richard A. Katz.

The process of flower essences starts with collecting the blossoms of plants, then placing the blossoms in a glass bowl of purified water and infusing in the direct sun for several hours.

Once the plant matter is filtered out, the process requires further dilution, potentizing (rhythmic shaking), and then preservation with either brandy or glycerite.

Hydrosols- Hydrosols are the aromatic waters created as a co-distillation during the steam distillation of essential oils or as a stand-alone product. The resulting product contains the water chemical components of the aromatic plants. Unlike essential oils, hydrosols are much safer when added to water, other beverages, salad dressings, and food. They are an excellent addition to facial spritzers, compresses, and are safer to use directly on the skin, especially with children and elders, than essential oils.

Hydrosols are similar to essential oils but are very different in chemical properties, shelf life, precautions, usage, and storage.

Basic Differences of Hydrosols and Essential Oils

- Hydrosols are water-based. Essential oils are lipid-based.
- Hydrosols have a shorter shelf-life and are best kept refrigerated.
- Hydrosols can become easily contaminated by bacteria. Essential oils can become oxidized.
- Hydrosols are not as concentrated as an essential oil, and most can be used undiluted on the skin.

Essential Oils- The oils from aromatic plants that are extracted from steam distillation, cold pressing, CO_2 (Carbon Dioxide Extracts), and solvent extraction (absolutes). These extracted oils are a highly concentrated hydrophobic liquid containing volatile aroma compounds from aromatic plants. This is a unique and relatively newer form of plant medicine than the extensive history of herbology. Aromatics that were utilized during ancient times were crude solvent extractions using fats and pressed oils. They were not very concentrated and contained very different chemistry than the essential oils of today. Qualitative research and long-term effects of distilled essential oils have only been documented within the last 100 years.

Essential oils do have tremendous effects on many systems of the body, including the limbic system, which is a very unique benefit of this particular herbal modality.

Methods of Extraction

The use of aromatic plant extracts and essential oils has been embraced by civilizations for thousands of years. Through crude extraction methods, ancient cultures derived aromatic oils from seeds, roots, bark, leaves, wood, flowers, and resins and used them in religious ceremony, perfumery, funerary services, and many other aspects of life. In the early Orient, Greece and Rome, the aromatic oils were obtained by placing plant material into a fatty oil, leaving them to warm in the sun and finally separating out the aromatic components.

Today, there are several methods of plant extraction. Steam distillation is the most widely used process for extraction on a large scale and is the standard method for producing essential oils. CO_2 extracts are oils similar to distilled essential oils and can be tremendously beneficial when used in aromatherapy. Solvent extraction methods produce absolutes, which are different from essential oils because they can contain both aromatic and non-aromatic chemical constituents.

Steam Distillation
Steam distillation causes sacs in plant material to open and release their oils, but this process can't extract heavier compounds, and some constituents can be damaged due to the high heat. Steam distillation of all aromatic plants can be done for both essential oils and hydrosols. There are many glass and copper home garden distillers on the market. They typically range in size from 2 to 300 liters. However, you will only get hydrosol from the smaller liter sizes. I have used glass, stainless steel, and copper stills and prefer the copper still because of the difference in the beautiful aroma and taste of the hydrosols produced from this still.

CO^2 Extracts

A relatively new, and highly efficient process, is CO^2 extraction. The process consists of pumping pressurized carbon dioxide into a chamber filled with plant matter. When carbon dioxide is subjected to pressure it has liquid properties while remaining in a gaseous state. Because of these liquid properties, the carbon dioxide functions as a solvent, pulling the oils and other substances, such as pigment and resin, from the plant material.

The difference between CO^2 extraction and traditional steam distillation is that CO^2 is used as a solvent instead of heated water or steam.

Let's compare the differences in the two methods:

Steam Distillation

- Involves temperatures of around 140 to 212 degrees F.
- High heat changes the molecular composition of the plant.

CO^2 Extraction

- Temperatures of about 95 to 100 degrees F.
- Superior in many cases due to lower heat exposure of plant matter.
- The extracts contain more plant constituents.
- More full-bodied aroma, closely resembling the herb from which it is derived.

As this newer method of extraction becomes established in aromatherapy, more choices are emerging. Here is a look at several commonly CO^2 extracted oils and their uses:

Arnica Flower *(Arnica montana)* – With amazing anti-inflammatory actions, this extract is an excellent choice for salves and ointments for bruises. Also known to support healthy hair growth, one to two percent dilution can be added to hair care preparations.

Calendula *(Calendula officinalis)* – Most recognized for its ability to help wound healing, ulcers and abrasions. A CO^2 extract contains not only all the essential oils of the plant, but also the plant waxes and heavier phytochemicals. This extract can be used in healing salves, lotions, and creams for chapped, dry or damaged skin. Recommended to use one-to-five percent dilution in formulations.

Carrot Seed *(Daucus carota)* – This CO^2 is used primarily for its healing properties and its effects on the skin. It helps repair and tone the skin, increase elasticity, and reduces the formation of wrinkles and scars. An excellent addition to face creams, it is useful for balancing oily and dry skin. (Not for use during pregnancy or breastfeeding.)

Coffee Bean *(Coffea arabica L)* – The uplifting scent of this extract is the rich, warm, smooth aroma of fresh roasted coffee. Known to reduce puffiness, fine lines and wrinkles, it is a suitable choice for cosmetics, skin and body care products. This extract contains Cafestol, a diterpene, which is under study for its diverse pharmacological benefits. It is also used in perfumery and is considered a base note. (Contains 0.5% caffeine: avoid if sensitive.)

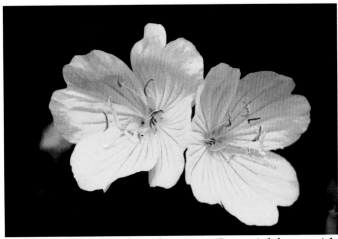

Evening Primrose *(Oenothera biennis)*
This CO^2 is naturally rich in gamma-linolenic essential fatty acid and is exceptionally nourishing to the skin.

Since the human body doesn't produce essential fatty acids, it's important to obtain them through nutrition and topical application. Essential fatty acids inhibit bacterial growth and defend against infection and inflammation. Evening Primrose is highly beneficial for dry skin problems including eczema and psoriasis.

Ginger *(Zingiber officinale)* – A ginger CO^2 has a very warm, spicy and more complex aroma than that of the distilled essential oil. This should be used sparingly due to its intensity. Dilute and add gradually to blends until the desired effect is achieved. It is especially well suited for natural perfumery to introduce warmth and a spicy sweetness. (Not for use in the bath or those with sensitive skin.)

Jasmine *(Jasminum sambac)* – An uplifting aroma which encourages a focused mind. Jasmine CO^2 possesses a very rich, floral aroma that is wonderful in perfumes. The aroma is quite concentrated, and a little goes a very long way. Dilute in Jojoba to fragrance your most special formulations. (Not suggested for children under 5 years.)

Vanilla *(Vanilla planifolia)* – Vanilla CO^2 extract is usually added to blends to help sweeten, soften and deepen the fragrance. Suitable for all ages and genders. The rich aroma blends especially well with essential oils and other natural aromatics in the spice, citrus, mint, herbaceous and wood categories.

CO^2 extraction produces the most therapeutic oil from many plants, but not all. It is highly beneficial for resins such as Frankincense *(Boswellia carterii)* and Myrrh *(Commiphora myrrha)* as more of the heavier compounds, and important healing properties, are included in the finished product.

CO^2 extraction can be important when rare or endangered plant species are involved, such as Sandalwood *(Santalum album)*, since less of the plant is needed to produce an equivalent amount of oil.

Absolutes

Absolutes offer a wonderful way to capture floral fragrances more accurately. They differ from essential oils in that they contain not only essential oil, but also a higher density of coloring, waxes, and other constituents from the plant.

The efficiency and low temperature of this particular extraction process helps to prevent damage to the fragrant compounds. Most absolutes carry the aromas closest to the original plant than is possible with essential oils produced through steam distillation.

Absolutes are used extensively in the cosmetic and perfume industries due to their strong aromas.

Absolutes do require the use of solvent extraction techniques or, more traditionally, enfleurage.

Solvent extraction is used on plant material that is more delicate and not easily steam distilled. One example is tuberose *(Polianthes tuberosa)*. If it was steam distilled, very little oil would be produced, and the oil would not have as nice an aroma as solvent extracted tuberose.

Solvent extraction is used for jasmine *(Jasminum sambac)*, tuberose *(Polianthes tuberosa)*, carnation *(Dianthus caryophyllus)*, gardenia *(Gardenia jasminoides)*, mimosa *(Albizia julibrissin)*, violet leaf *(Viola odorata)* and other delicate flowers. Others, like neroli *(Citrus aurantium var. amara)* and rose *(Rosa damascena)*, can be either steam distilled or solvent-extracted.

Also, some raw materials are either too delicate or too inert to be steam-distilled and can only yield their aroma through other methods, such as solvent extraction or lipid absorption.

Acquiring an absolute is a multi-step process:

First step: Extracting the aromatic oil from the plant material with a chemical solvent such as hexane or toluene. After the solvent is removed, what is left behind is a waxy substance called a concrete or resinoid, depending on if the extract is waxy or resinous. Concretes and resinoids are used in a wide range of industries, but specialist knowledge is required to use them because they are very difficult to work with due to their thick, heavy consistency. This is one of the main reasons that concretes and resinoids with the exception of benzoin *(Styrax benzoin)* are rarely used in aromatherapy.

Second step: The aromatic oils are then extracted from the concrete with ethyl alcohol to separate the aromatic compounds from pigments and waxes. Many of these waxes have little aromatic value and make the oil challenging to use due to their insolubility, although these waxes are useful in skin care products.

After the ethyl alcohol is removed, the remaining substance is an absolute, an oil with an aroma close to the plant from which it came.

An absolute is the most concentrated form of fragrance and highly regarded in natural perfumery.

Once the solvent extraction process has been completed, the resulting absolute will have an extremely low concentration of solvent residue, approximately five to ten ppm (parts per million). In the past, there were concerns related to the solvent and alcohol residues left in absolutes, which were claimed to be unacceptably high for use in aromatherapy. "However, this issue dates back to the late 1950's when this process was still in its infancy and quality standards were a great deal lower, as pointed out by experts at that time, such as Steffen Arctander *(Perfume and Flavour Materials of Natural Origin,* 1961)."[1]

Rest assured that since solvents are very expensive, the manufacturers are more enthusiastic to recapture every last drop for recycling. There is no reason for them to leave residues of any kind in the product. The analytical testing of gas chromatography and mass spectrometry (GC/MS) also reveals unwanted residues.

Absolutes are generally much more concentrated than essential oils. While it is true that a little essential oil goes a long way, a little absolute goes an even longer way. Because of their high concentration absolutes are often used in aromatherapy perfumery. Absolutes can also be blended with other essential oils, CO^2 extracts, and herbal infusions.

Through my personal and professional use of herbs, flower essences, essential oils, CO^2s, absolutes, and hydrosols, over several decades, I have concluded that herbs, flower essences, and some hydrosols are best to use internally. Applications of essential oils, CO^2s, and absolutes are best used externally. Particularly in the United States, there is much controversy and misinformation about the use of essential oils taken internally. When you look at the relatively short history of the use of essential oils compared to herbs, there is not enough verified research that definitively states the long-term safety of ingestion of essential oils. For many reasons, I assert that using herbs internally is much more beneficial.

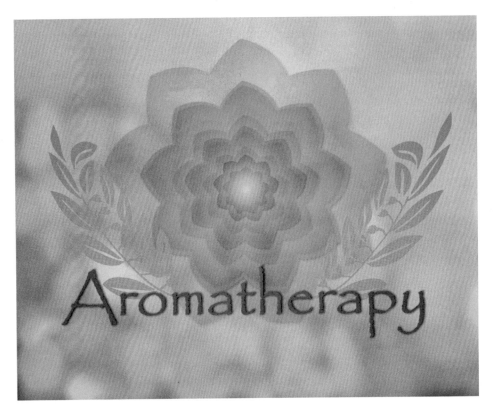

Aromatherapy

One of the distinct characteristics of aromatherapy, as a natural healing modality, is the vast variety of applications that can be utilized. Many products can be formulated using various combinations of essential oils, carrier oils, infusions, flower essences, and hydrosols.

Uses of Essential Oils:

- Diffusing
- Nasal inhaler or aroma patch
- Room or facial spritzer
- Shower spritzer
- Dead Sea salt shower scrub
- Bath
- Compresses
- Body oil or lotion
- Salve
- Massage oils
- Added to personal care products
- Household cleaning products

These options allow you to choose the application method(s) that are best suited to your needs. Let's take a brief look at the various aromatherapy application methods.

Inhalation Applications: Inhalation is the easiest and most direct method for essential oils to enter the limbic system in the brain. Inhalation can be done through various methods: by direct inhalation of essential oils from a cotton ball, or tissue; steam inhalation; diffusers; and through the use of personal nasal inhalers.

The easiest inhalation application is on a tissue or cotton ball. Add two to three drops of essential oil to a tissue or cotton ball, place near your nose and inhale deeply several times.

Diffusing: Follow the instructions of use for the particular type of diffuser you own. Add 15 to 25 drops of an essential oil or a blend to the diffuser.

One of my favorite diffuser blends: equal drops of Sweet Orange *(Citrus sinensis)*, Coriander *(Coriandrum sativum)*, and Black Spruce *(Picea mariana)*.

Personal Nasal Inhaler: Excellent to use for sinus and respiratory issues, mental relaxation, or to enhance mental focus or relaxation. No carrier oil is needed with a personal inhaler.

Place the cotton wick in a small glass bowl and then add a blend of 15 to 25 drops essential oil. Allow the cotton wick to absorb all of the essential oils. Insert the cotton wick into the nasal inhaler and snap the bottom shut.

Examples of a nasal inhaler blend:

Relaxing Blend: Equal drops of **cypress** *(Cupressus sempervirens)*, **mandarin** *(Citrus reticulata)*, and **vetiver** *(Vetiveria zizanoides)*.

Stimulating Blend: Saturate the nasal inhaler wick with these stimulating essential oils:

- 6 drops of **rosemary** *(Rosmarinus officinalis)*
- 6 drops of **basil** *(Ocimum basilicum)*
- 4 drops **peppermint** *(Mentha piperita)*

This blend is very stimulating, best to stop using this inhaler four to six hours before sleep.

Aroma Patch

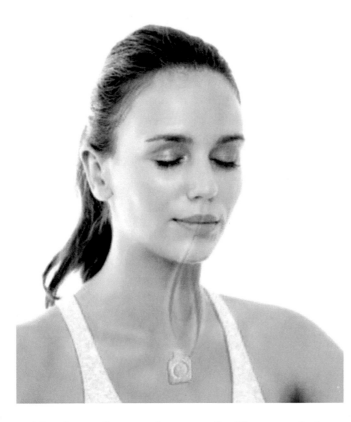

These small 1″x1″ patches are perfect to wear in a "no scents" environment like school, work, hospitals, nursing homes, or while traveling.

Pre-made Aroma Patches are available that have essential oils that are perfect to use for general stress relief, anxiety, fatigue, respiratory complaints, nausea, and insomnia.

There are also blank patches that you can load two to three drops of a single essential oil or a blend into the round receptacle. Then, apply it to your collarbone, upper chest or apply to the inside of your shirt to allow the vapor to reach your nose.

The patch allows for a sustained release of the essential oil molecules, lasting approximately six to eight hours. The Aromatherapy Inhalation Patch uses a patented technology featuring an FDA approved medical adhesive. These can be safely applied directly to the skin or on clothing.

Steam Inhalation: Add three to five drops of essential oil to a steaming bowl of hot water, then cover your head with a towel, close your eyes and bend over the steaming bowl of water using the towel as a tent to trap the steam. Deeply inhale for several minutes.

Steam inhalation can be used as a facial steam or for opening the sinuses and respiratory system.

Topical Applications: Enables the healing benefits of essential oils to be absorbed into the blood stream through the skin. Topical application also combines the benefits of essential oils with the benefits of carrier oils. When you are applying a topical blend keep in mind the system(s) of the body you are trying to affect. It does not make sense to increase circulation to the legs by applying the blend to your wrists or the bottoms of your feet. Think about the areas of the physical body that are in pain, inflamed or in need of re-education to reach a state of balance.

Essential oil dilution ratios for topical blends:

- 0.5-1% dilution = Six drops essential oil per one-ounce carrier oil. Use for children, elders, during pregnancy, and individuals with weakened systems and/or sensitivities.
- 2% dilution = Twelve drops essential oil per one-ounce carrier oil. Use for general, whole body massage.
- 3% dilution = Eighteen drops essential oil per one-ounce carrier oil. Use for localized massage, acute conditions and those with higher metabolisms.

General areas to apply an aromatherapy blend for topical application:

Respiratory issues: Apply to the neck, upper chest, upper back, shoulders, and across the bridge of the nose for sinus issues.

Digestive issues: Massage the abdomen in a clockwise fashion. Also massage from the throat to the pelvis, as well as the mid to lower back.

Hormonal issues: Upper chest, abdomen, on the back from the kidneys to the sacrum, and around the hips.

Circulatory issues: Apply to the chest, abdomen, and legs.

Bone, joint, and muscle inflammation: Apply to the specific areas of pain, as well as the corresponding areas on the spine.

Bathing Applications: Bathing with essential oils can include the use of bath salts, bath blends, and soaps. Bathing provides several methods for the healing benefits of essential oils to enter the body, including by absorption through the skin and inhalation of the bath steam.

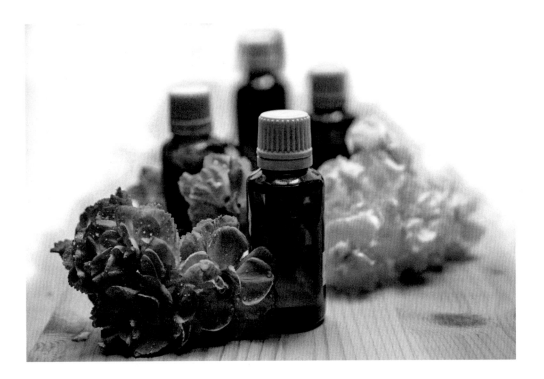

Bath Blends: Add five to ten drops of essential oil to one tablespoon of jojoba (*Simmondsia chinensis*), castile soap, or Solubol*, stir well and then add to the bath water before stepping into the tub. Remember to avoid all skin irritating essential oils including, citrus oils.

*For those with a bee sensitivity or allergy, please note that some formulations of Solubol do contain beeswax and bee propolis.

Bath Salts: Add five to ten drops of essential oil to one tablespoon of carrier oil, like jojoba (*Simmondsia chinensis*), stir and then add blend to one to two cups of Epsom or Dead Sea salts. Add the bath salts to the bath water before stepping into the tub. Remember to avoid all skin irritating essential oils including citrus oils.

Shower Scrubs: These are useful to increase circulation and lymphatic movement, and reduce inflammation, exfoliate the skin, relieve pain and discomfort. To avoid dermal abrasion, use fine grain Dead Sea salt or regular sea salt. Carrier oils, such as Safflower *(Carthamus tinctorius),* and essential oils are also used in a shower scrub.

Add five to ten drops of essential oil to two to three tablespoons of carrier oil, stir and add this blend to 1/4 cup fine grain Dead Sea salt and 1/4 cup regular sea salt. In a dry shower, gently massage your body in long smooth strokes toward the heart (subclavian vein) and then rinse off in the shower.

I prefer using salts in scrubs rather than sugar because salt also cleanses the energy field.

Compresses: Add three to six drops of essential oil to one-tablespoon of carrier oil or Solubol, and then add the blend to either hot or cold compress water. Aromatherapy compresses help to ease and reduce the swelling, pain, and stiffness of muscles and joints, or the discomfort of bruises.

When formulating an aromatherapy blend I hope you refer to these easy to follow instructions, because by doing so you are using the power of essential oils in the safest and most beneficial manner.

Aromatherapy can also be easily integrated into many other healing modalities:

- Massage/bodywork
- Acupressure
- Acupuncture
- Chiropractic
- Naturopathy
- Shiatsu
- Cranial Sacral
- Reflexology
- Energy Medicine: like Pranic Healing, Reiki, and Medical Qigong
- Emotional Freedom Techniques (EFT), also known as Tapping

Chapter 4

Seasonal Wellness

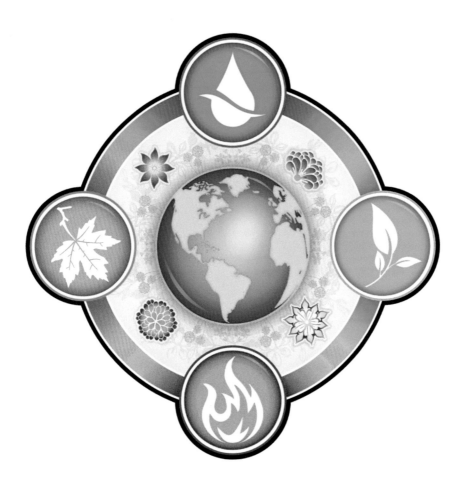

Many journeys of self-discovery take place around a traumatic event. My inner healing journey began with the death of my mother when I was fourteen. She had a gallbladder operation and ended up getting septic poisoning and passed within twenty-four hours. This traumatic event was an extreme turning point in my life. She had always been there for me as an excellent mother. She was very kind, compassionate, and loving. It took more than twenty years to get over her death and feel stable on my own. After that life-changing experience, I connected with the Earth and spirit as my mother. The Earth was my grounding and comfort, and has guided me through my life.

At seventeen I graduated high school six months early and went straight into college. At that time I attended three different colleges. The one best-suited for me was Evergreen State College in Olympia, Washington. I studied in a program called Human Health and Behavior, which included all of the "ologies" related to anatomy, physiology, neurology, psychology, sociology, massage training, and a counseling internship. I also gave my first presentations on the acupressure meridians and reflexology. I realized, at that point, instead of just talking to people I needed to be able to incorporate healing touch. This was the beginning of my journey into becoming a practitioner of bodywork and holistic healing. It has been a fascinating journey, realizing that we are more than just a physical body and how the body, mind, spirit, and emotions all work intricately together to support human life.

I went on to study for the next ten years with Lar Short, a dynamic teacher of Total Person Facilitation, which is an integrative approach to working with the body, mind, and spirit. My travels also took me to Thailand to study with Master Mantak Chia, who teaches Taoist alchemy, and what is called "Chi Nei Tsang", a system of hands-on abdominal healing.

For me, one of the exciting aspects of working with the internal organs was recognizing how emotions can get stagnate and congested in the internal organs, which could end up causing different types of dis-ease. For example, feelings of anger, resentment, and jealousy can affect the liver and gallbladder in a harmful way. Fortunately, there is also the positive, or virtuous, side of the energy, which, to me, is the ultimate expression of grace and healing within our lives. The virtues of the liver are kindness and forgiveness.

I also spent seven years traveling and studying with Native American medicine tribes of the Lakota, Navajo, and Pima. I was even spiritually adopted into a Navajo family. The medicine men, in particular, were intricately involved in connecting with the elements. These fantastic experiences created a three-pronged healing foundation that I have continued to nurture with the seasonal elements; which has assisted me to live my life in harmony, to become a more loving and compassionate person, and to be aware of imbalances before they become dis-ease. I am so grateful for the opportunities to be with these teachers.

These experiences had a tremendous impact on my life's journey and assisted me in profoundly integrating the seasonal elements within myself. Giving me very precise information on the connections with my body, mind, spirit, and emotions and how to live my daily life in harmony, encouraging a healthy radiance.

As you have your own inner journey, a good question to ask yourself is, "How can I connect deeper with nature and my innate healing wisdom"?

Because of my experience working with different forms of seasonal healing, I have a fascination with nature's cycles and how these cycles correspond with human life in different cultures.

In the Native American perspective, Earth is at the center, surrounded by the four directions:

- South - Summer
- West- Autumn
- North- Winter
- East- Spring

In the Ayurvedic perspective, there is the seasonal division of:

- Pitta- Summer
- Kapha - Autumn and Early winter
- Vata- Second half of Winter and Spring

From my studies, I have found that the Chinese five element theory, or phases, is the most detailed and has many correspondences to seasons, colors, internal organs, emotional imbalances, and dis-eased states. The elements represented in this perspective are Wood, Fire, Earth, Metal, and Water.

The seasons can also correspond to our human life cycles:

- Spring- Birth
- Summer - Growth- Adolescence
- Late Fall - Maturity
- Fall- Harvest - Retirement
- Winter- Restoration - Death

Personally, this information has been tremendously useful in guiding me throughout my adult life, and as an awareness to living in a balanced and healthy state of being. The next chapters in this book will integrate many healing modalities for each season of the year. Enjoy the journey!

Grounding and Centering Your Earth Element

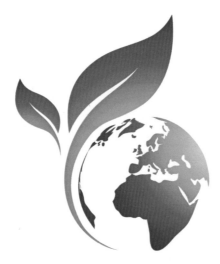

For me, I feel the Earth element is balanced when I am grounded and centered, connected to my body, mind, spirit, emotions, and environment.

The Earth Element symbolizes the center, balance, and groundedness. It is the axis of the elements, mandala or medicine wheel: the point where we stand looking out at the four cardinal directions. Earth phase corresponds to the center, the middle, the balance between Yang and Yin. Earth energy is stable, giving us a firm center and a grounding presence.

In the element theory of healing, it relates to late summer, or the in-between season, before autumn starts. This time is the peak to harvest plants, the time of ripening fruit and grains, and when the energy begins to wane; becoming more cooling in the evenings, and when the first golden leaves start to appear on the trees.

Days and nights are nearly equal in length. The climate is perfect – neither too hot nor too cold, neither to wet nor too dry.

There are many different aspects and characteristics of the Earth element. Let's start with the beautiful bright yellow or amber color. The color amber is similar to the golden color of grain right before harvest and similar to dried sap from a tree. Both have a sweet and grounding scent, which reminds me of one of my favorite essential oils, Vetiver *(Vetiveria zizanoides)*.

In my experience, Earth energy is ALL about grounding and centering.
To ground means you are focused and clear, that you are well balanced, make sensible choices for yourself, and have proper personal boundaries. Over the years, I have found that grounding meditation and exercise have been beneficial in keeping me connected to the Earth element.

To activate grounding and centering, move your body! Yoga, tai chi, qigong, massage, foot reflexology, acupressure, and walking in nature are all very beneficial for connecting deeper with the Earth element. I prefer Hatha yoga, in which the movements are slower and the poses are held longer, which allows the fascia, the connective tissue, to open up and stretch. This allows time for integrating and releasing held emotions or contraction within the bodymind, which will aid in grounding.

Get your feet on the ground!

Envision your legs like tree trunks rooted to the Earth. Your feet and legs are your grounding cords or your "roots." Like a plant's root system, you also have a grounding cord to stabilize you, so that whatever happens you can remain stable in the grounded energy of the Earth.

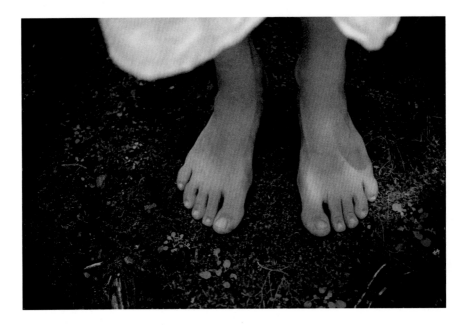

The human species evolved in the forests. As we have become more modern and drifted away from nature into urbanization, we seem to have left the serenity of touching the earth back in the forests. In the 1980's the Japanese developed Shinrin-yoku which means, "taking in the forest atmosphere," or "forest bathing," as a way to connect with the Earth element.

In California, there is the Association of Nature & Forest Therapy. Melanie Chouckas-Bradley is certified as a forest therapy guide. She explains that the aim of forest bathing is to slow down and become immersed in the natural environment. Activation of the senses during forest bathing is a time to connect with the smells, textures, tastes, and sights of the forest.

You can practice this centering awareness anywhere in nature. Simply take in the feelings and sounds of your environment, allowing your awareness to expand as your senses open.

**"The clearest way into the Universe is through a forest wilderness."
John Muir**

Abdominal breathing is also a very effective way to stabilize the core of your being.

Slow abdominal breathing reduces the "fight-or-flight" response of the sympathetic nervous system. A relaxation response is created when we relax our abdomen and pelvic diaphragm. Draw in a deep abdominal breath, allowing the breath to fill the lungs from the bottom to the top of the thorax while expanding the belly and chest in a coordinated sequence. This process creates a parasympathetic nervous system toning. This type of breathing is called the "relaxing breath," or "the calming breath." It is best to keep your focus and attention on your abdomen while you breathe.

Abdominal Brain

The Earth element also has a potent effect on the digestive process, the center of our body. This element is connected with the internal organs of the stomach, spleen, and pancreas, which transport nourishment.

In 1984, I started studying the bodymind therapy of Chi Nei Tsang, a detoxifying and energizing abdominal massage. This type of healing bodywork was the beginning of my ten-year study and teachers training in this healing modality. I realized how acute the function of the abdomen is to our overall health, as it is the center of our body and the engine. I have found that when I am aware of my digestion, lower my stress levels, practice deep abdominal breathing, eat highly nutritious foods, and include digestive enzymes and probiotics, everything else in my body and mind is healthier and happier.

In the book review of *The Good Gut: Taking Control of Your Weight, Your Mood and Your Long-Term Health*, Justin Sonnenburg, Ph.D. and Erica Sonnenburg, Ph.D., express, "A primal connection exists between our brain and our gut. We often talk about a "gut feeling" when we meet someone for the first time. We're told to "trust our gut instinct" when making a difficult decision, or that it's "gut check time" when faced with a situation that tests our nerve and determination. This mind-gut connection is not just metaphorical.

Our brain and gut are connected by an extensive network of neurons, and a highway of chemicals and hormones that constantly provide feedback about how hungry we are, whether or not we're experiencing stress, or if we've ingested a disease-causing microbe. This information superhighway is called the "brain-gut axis," and it provides constant updates on the state of affairs at your two ends." [1]

Upon further research, I found a fascinating article by Henry A. Nasrallah, MD, called *Psychoneurogastroenterology: The abdominal brain, the microbiome, and psychiatry*. Nasrallah states, " Over the last decade there is substantial evidence of a gastrointestinal (GI) nervous system, which is different and distinct from the Central Nervous System (CNS) that comprises the brain and spinal cord. This has been recognized for more than a century, but it seems that the western medical community has generally ignored it. This nervous system is located inside the wall of the GI tract, extending from the esophagus to the rectum. Technically, it is known as the enteric nervous system or ENS, but it has been given other labels, too: "second brain," "abdominal brain," "other brain," and "back-up brain." The Enteric Brain is located in the sheets of cells lining the esophagus, stomach, small intestines, and large intestines. It is considered to be a separate entity unto itself because even if you cut all the nerves running to the Enteric Brain, it could still function independently. This second brain is composed of a network of different kinds of neurons, neurotransmitters, and proteins that carry messages between other neurons, interneurons, and immune cells.

The Enteric Brain contains 100 million neurons more than the spinal cord. Significate neurotransmitters, such as serotonin, dopamine, glutamate, and norepinephrine, are found in the Enteric Brain. 95% of the body's serotonin, best known as the anti-depressive or ecstasy molecule, is located here, along with significant cells of the immune system's inflammatory network."[2]

In 1999, Dr. Michael Gershon wrote an amazing book called, *The Second Brain: A Groundbreaking New Understanding of Nervous Disorders of the Stomach and Intestine*. In the description of the book it notes: " Dr. Michael Gershon has devoted his career to understanding the human bowel (the stomach, esophagus, small intestine, and colon). His thirty years of research have led to an extraordinary rediscovery: nerve cells in the gut that act as a brain. This "second brain" can control our gut all by itself. Our two brains -- the one in our head and the one in our bowel -- must cooperate. If they do not, then there is chaos in the gut and misery in the head -- everything from "butterflies" to cramps, from diarrhea to constipation.

Dr. Gershon's work has led to radical new understandings about a wide range of gastrointestinal problems including gastroenteritis, nervous stomach, and irritable bowel syndrome. The Second Brain represents a quantum leap in medical knowledge and is already benefiting patients whose symptoms were previously dismissed as neurotic or, "it's all in your head," diagnosis."[3]

For me, Dr. Gershon's research suggests that when the abdominal brain is out of balance, it can create systemic inflammation, an imbalance which can also affect our attitude, moods, and general outlook on life. Using methods of positive autonomic nervous system stimulation balances the Enteric Brain function. This conclusion represents a significant change in understanding the value of therapeutic healing approaches and has the potential to end a large amount of human suffering and disease.

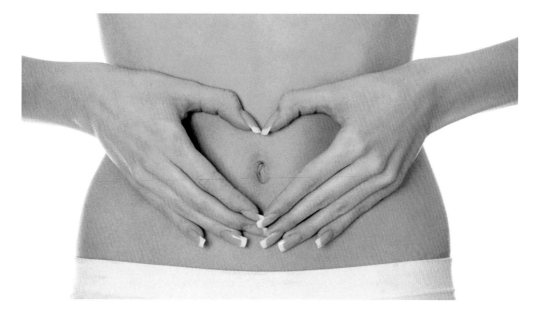

If you experience digestive issues on a regular basis consider these basic suggestions:

- Sit down to eat, not on the go.
- Choose highly nutritious foods that are organic and unprocessed.
- Eat slowly and mindfully with each bite.
- Only drink a small amount of warm beverages during your meal. Cold drinks dramatically reduce the digestive activity.
- Do not eat when you are emotionally charged.
- The use of digestive supplements and probiotics.

There are beneficial herbal uses for each season of the year to promote a robust immune system, reduce emotional distress, and establish a sense of ease in the bodymind and spirit. The next section in this chapter will recommend herbs, flower essences, hydrosols, essential oils and applications for the earth element.

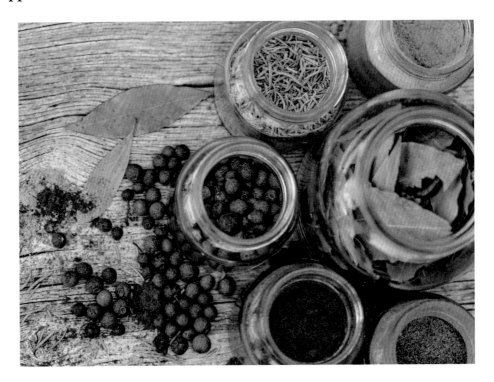

Earth Herbs

Spices have been used throughout history to increase the digestive process.

Historically, culinary spices and herbs were used as food preservatives and also for their digestive and health-enhancing properties. Some of these spices are used best as tea, powdered for capsules, and cooking. A few of these spices and herbs include; black pepper *(Piper nigrum)*, caraway *(Carum carvi)*, cardamom *(Elettaria cardamomum)*, cinnamon *(Cinnamomum zeylanicum)*, clove *(Syzygium aromaticum)*, coriander *(Coriandrum sativum)*, cumin *(Cuminum cyminum)*, fennel *(Foeniculum vulgare)*, garlic *(Allium sativum)*, ginger *(Zingiber officinale)*, thyme *(Thymus vulgaris)* and turmeric *(Curcuma longa)*.

These spices not only add delicious flavor to food, but are also known to increase digestion, reduce inflammation, and increase immunity.

There are many digestive and immune stimulating herbs that can be used in cooking, teas, or taken in capsules.

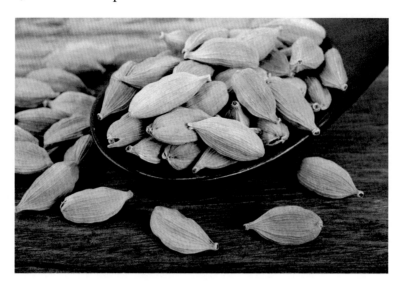

Cardamom (*Elettaria cardamomum*)

The green variety of cardamom originates from India to Malaysia.
This herb is used abundantly in Asian cooking for both sweet and savory dishes.

It is a wonderful herb that settles digestion, heartburn, intestinal spasms, relieves flatulence, diarrhea, constipation, liver and gallbladder complaints, and loss of appetite.

Cardamom adds a spicy warmth to Chai Tea.

Enjoy this Chai Tea recipe from *The Way of Herbs* by Michael Tierra.

Simmer the following herbs in one quart of water:

- 1oz. of sliced or grated fresh ginger
- seven peppercorns
- one cinnamon stick
- five cloves
- fifteen cardamom seeds

After fifteen minutes add one-half cup of milk, simmer for another ten minutes. Add a sprinkle of nutmeg and a few drops of vanilla extract.

Drink one cup of tea, sweetened with honey, twice per day or as needed for warmth and digestion.

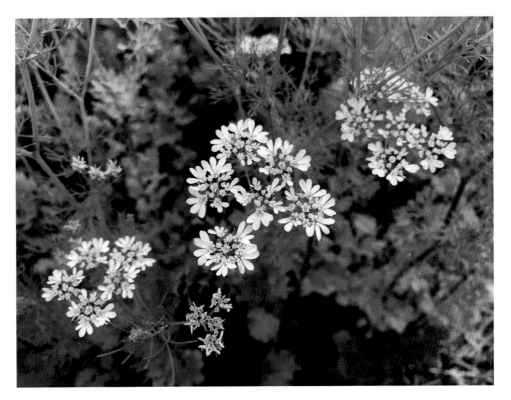

Cilantro/ Coriander *(Coriandrum sativum)* - Did you know that these two herbs come from the same plant? Cilantro is from the leaves and coriander is from the seeds.

Cilantro herb is a wonderful addition in teas, soups and salads, or blended into salad dressings. It acts as a general cleanser of the body, to rid it of toxins and fluid wastes. This herb is excellent for adding to soups, Asian dishes, and tea.

Coriander seed is used to relieve mental fatigue. It has a warming and tonic effect on the digestive and glandular systems. The seed is also excellent in soups, Asian food, and teas.

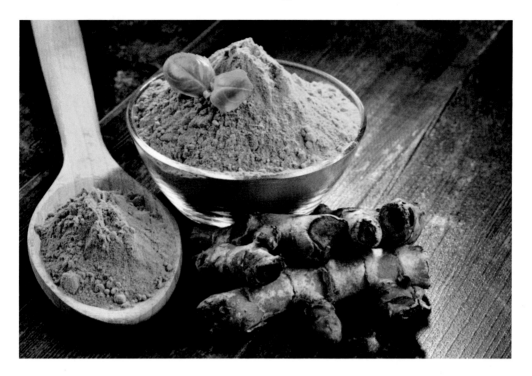

Turmeric *(Curcuma longa)*
This plant is from the Zingiberaceae family, and is a relative of ginger (*Zingiber officinale*). You may be familiar with turmeric, as it is used as the main spice in curry.

Turmeric is widely used in cooking and gives Indian curry its flavor and yellow color. It is also used in mustard and to color butter and cheese.

Turmeric contains curcumin, which is a powerful antioxidant. This antioxidant is an excellent scavenger of free radicals, which can damage cell membranes and even cause cell death. Antioxidants can fight free radicals and may reduce, or help prevent, some of the damage they cause.

Turmeric root has been used in both Ayurvedic and Chinese medicine as an anti-inflammatory, to reduce digestive and liver problems, skin issues, wounds, and a variety of other inflammatory issues.

According to a fabulous article by Edward F. Block, published in the International Journal of Complementary & Alternative Medicine, "Turmeric by itself is not very well absorbed by the small intestinal mucosa. However, if you mix turmeric with black pepper, the absorption increases by 1000 times better! Combine turmeric powder with equal amounts of freshly ground black pepper in olive oil and add to a stir-fry, soup, or stew."[4]

Earth Flower Essences

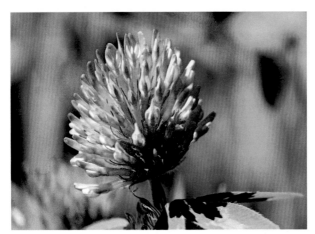

Red Clover
(Trifolium pretense)

Red Clover flower essence helps to encourage a sense of individuality and self-awareness, encourages a calm self-acceptance connected to a deeper knowing.

Encourages Positive Qualities:
Self-awareness
Self-confidence
Steady and calm abiding
"Centered Self-Awareness"

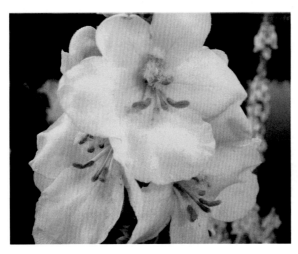

Mullein *(Verbascum thapsus)*
Mullein assists in self-acceptance and awareness of one's inner worth and values. Useful for those who experience depression, fear, abandonment, sadness, irritability, and anxiety. Revitalizes intimacy in relationships.
Reaffirms focus and purpose for those who have lost their direction.

Encourages Positive Qualities:
Sense of protection
Emotional self-nurturance
Calming and comforting
Knowing vulnerability as strength
"Calm Acceptance"

Earth Hydrosol

Frankincense *(Boswellia carterii)* – the aroma of the hydrosol is sweeter than the essential oil; the taste can be bitter if undiluted. This hydrosol soothes, relaxes, and reduces anxiety, opens the lungs, and is a beautiful addition to meditation practice. Excellent for skin care; facial toners, spritzers, and aftershave.

Earth Essential Oils are sweet, warming, and earthy with a deep rich scent.

- **Davana** *(Artemisia pallens)* - sweet and warming, increases immunity, clears internal dampness, reduces menstrual and menopausal complaints,
  calms the nerves and mind.
- **Sandalwood** *(Santalum spicatum)* - cooling, soothing for the mind, and emotions.
- **Vetiver** *(Vetiveria zizanoides)* - clears heat, increases immunity, calms nerves, and settles the mind.

Because of their depth of aroma, I experience absolutes as very centering; perfect for grounding the earth energy.

There are many amazing absolutes available to include in formulating your aromatherapy perfumes and colognes:

Beeswax *(Apis mellifera)*
Cassie *(Acacia farnesiana)*
Cocoa *(Theobroma cacao)*
Coffee Bean *(Coffea arabica)*
Jasmine *(Jasminum sambac)*

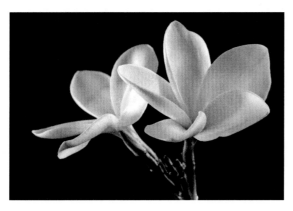

Frangipani *(Plumeria alba)*
Neroli *(Citrus aurantium var. amara)*
Rose *(Rosa damascena)*
Mimosa *(Acacia mirensi)*
Oakmoss *(Evernia prunastri)*
Osmanthus *(Osmanthus fragrans)*
Tuberose *(Polianthes tuberosa)*
Vanilla *(Vanilla planifolia)*
Violet Leaf *(Viola odorata)*

Here is one of my perfume blends that includes absolutes:

In a small ceramic bowl pour in 8mls of organic jojoba oil (*Simmondsia chinensis*).

Then, mix into the oil:

- **6 drops jasmine absolute** (*Jasminum sambac*)
- **3 drops tuberose absolute** (*Polianthes tuberosa*)
- **3 drops vanilla absolute** (*Vanilla planifolia*)
- **9 drops cardamom** (*Elettaria cardamomum*)
- **7 drops cypress** (*Cupressus sempervirens*)
- **5 drops rose geranium** (*Pelargonium roseum*)

Use a small funnel to load the blend into a 10ml roller bottle. Top off the remaining space with jojoba (*Simmondsia chinensis*). Shake well.

NOTE: This is a substantial perfume dilution and is just intended to be used in small dabs at a time. It is not recommended for children.

Enjoy this beautiful aromatic perfume!

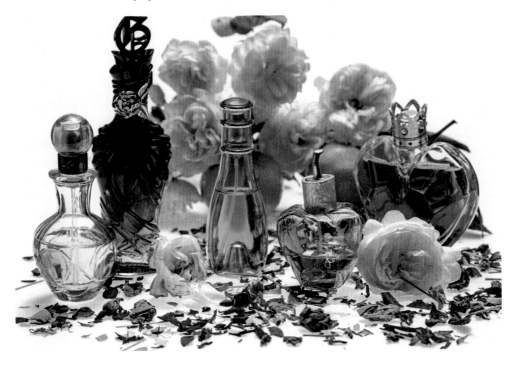

Earth Holistic Therapies

All the various types of massage and bodywork that were previously mentioned in Chapter Two are excellent for grounding and centering your bodymind. My favorite treatments for rooting myself and connecting deeper are reflexology and deep tissue with hot stones.

One of my favorite acupressure points for grounding is Kidney 1, also aptly known as the "Bubbling Spring" point. It is the first point on the kidney meridian and is the only acupressure point located on the bottom of the feet. You can easily stimulate this point by yourself, by sitting on the floor with your feet facing each other, or if you are sitting in a chair, you can bend your leg over the opposite thigh and work one foot at a time.

Benefits of Stimulating Kidney 1- Bubbling Spring

- Grounding
- Centering
- Calms anxiety
- Reduces headaches
- Reduces insomnia
- Reduces hot flashes and night sweats

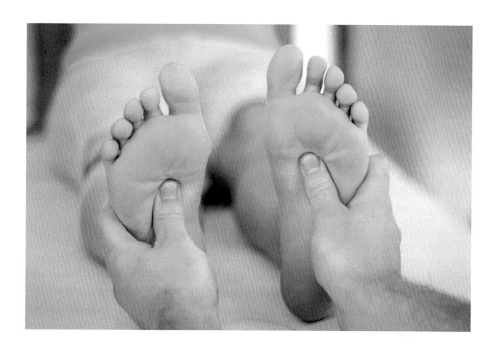

Earth Element Summary

As we continually nourish our grounding, it sustains our ability to move confidently for ourselves and into the world. Change is inevitable. The more we are rooted, the more focused and clear we will be to make wise choices. Establishing natural healing takes an interconnectedness with our body, mind, and spirit.

"Feeling rooted in the earth is soothing to the body, and it is our connection to the earth that gives us our most basic sense of belonging, home, resilience, and safety."
Jessica Moore

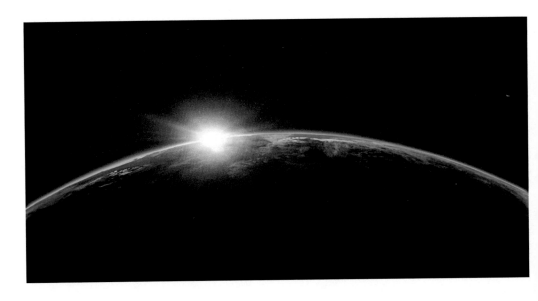

Chapter 5

Autumn

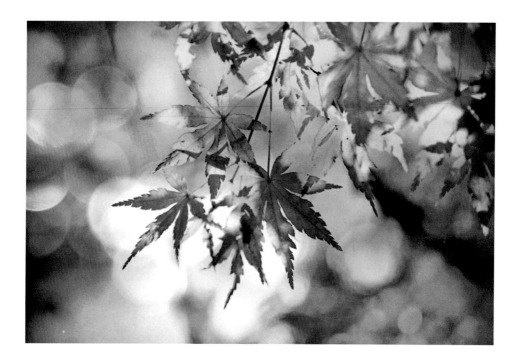

After the Autumn Equinox the weather turns cooler, and the nights are now longer than the days. The climate is drying, as leaves dry and fall from the trees. Coolness and darkness begin to predominate.

This time of year is contractive, moving in from all directions; we gather in our garden harvest, we begin to spend more time indoors, and we may start to become inwardly reflective. This element also represents the time of older adulthood and the beginning of our senior years, when our hair turns silvery and white. This season also corresponds to the direction of the West, and the time right after sunset.

When we are balanced during this season, we find ourselves well-organized, self-disciplined, methodical, discerning, reserved, precise, courageous, and conscientious. Beauty, ceremony, and refinement are revered.

If there are emotional imbalances, one may be taken over by grief and sadness, as well as becoming overly critical and having trouble letting go, expressing emotions, and being intimate. Physical imbalances are reflected in illnesses of the respiratory system and can also contribute to chronic constipation or other large intestine issues. The inherent dryness of this season can affect the skin; rashes, eczema, and different types of dry skin issues may be apparent.

When I find myself holding too much grief, sadness, or other disturbing

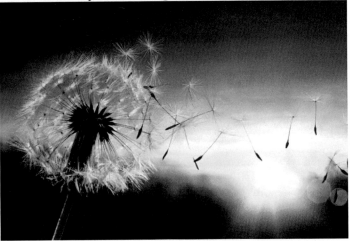

emotions, either from personal or worldly matters,
I let go of these mental constructs and come back to a sense of grace and ease within myself.

Sometimes a good cry will correct things very quickly. The tears, for me,

reflect the nourishing water that is cleansing. *Let it go~*

"To let go does not mean to get rid of. To let go means to let be.
When we let be with compassion, things come and go on their own."
Jack Kornfield

Autumn Herbs

These herbs can be used in the form of tea, decoction, infusion, or tincture.

Osha (*Ligusticum porteri*) - This root has been historically used as medicine by Native American and Hispanic cultures as an anti-viral for a sore throat, bronchitis, cough, common cold, influenza, and flu. It is also used to treat other viral infections including herpes and other immune deficiencies.

My personal experience with this fantastic root comes from when I was hiking in a high mountain region of Colorado. There was an overpowering scent of osha wafting in the area. When we pursued the origin of it we found beautiful osha plants and wild harvested a few roots. I was so enamored with the plant and the efficiency of its respiratory relief that I also named my first dog "Osha"!

Precautions: Osha is NOT advised during pregnancy or breastfeeding.

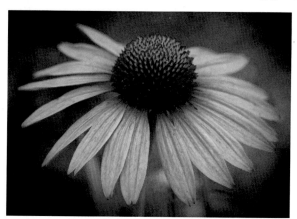

Echinacea (*Echinacea purpurea*) Used as 1st stage immune support. This herb reduces many symptoms of colds, flu, and infections. Michael Tierra states in his book, *The Way of Herbs,* "Echinacea is the wonder herb for all acute inflammatory conditions."[1]

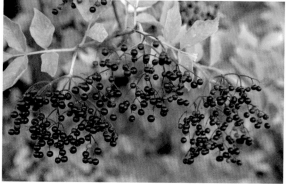

Elderberry (*Sambucus nigra*) Is an immune booster and an anti-bacterial berry that also decreases pain and inflammation. Good for colds, cases of flu and fevers, and reduces symptoms of upper respiratory infections. Elderberry syrup is an excellent choice for children, and it is such a tasty herbal remedy.

Directions of use: Follow label instructions. Generally, tinctures, are taken by the dropper full or added to water. A dropper equals approximately 30 drops.

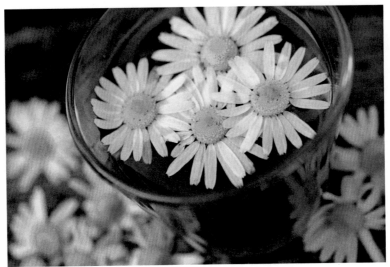

German Chamomile *(Matricaria recutita)* has a calming effect on the mind and body and is excellent in easing any inflammation.

The essential oil contains chamazulene, a potent anti-inflammatory chemical component. This blue chemical is not present in the plant, but forms in the distillation of the essential oil.

The fresh or dried flowers in a tea are excellent to use at nighttime for an insomnia remedy, to ensure a restful sleep. This herb is also an ingredient in "Sleepy Time Tea" from Celestial Seasonings. The hydrosol is very soothing for skin care and use with children.

Precautions: Avoid the use of German chamomile *(Matricaria recutita a.k.a Chamomilla recutita) essential oil* orally and with anti-coagulant medications.

Herbal Preparation for Autumn Plants

Drying Herbs- for culinary use or as herbal teas. After you harvest the plant materials, you can either place them in a basket with a cloth or paper towel in the bottom to soak up any moisture, hang them up, or put them into a paper bag.

Once they are well dried, put into a glass jar and label. It is best to store dried herbs in a dark and cool environment to prolong the shelf life. These dried herbs can be utilized throughout the year as tea, spices, infused oils, ground up for facial products, or distilled for hydrosols and essential oils.

 Infusion or Maceration is another method of extraction used for plants and herbs, typically used for non-aromatic plants. Although, I have successfully infused many dried aromatic plants from my botanical garden, including plants like German chamomile *(Matricaria recutita)*, Lavender *(Lavendula angustifolia)* and Yarrow *(Acheilia millefolium)*.

Examples of Infused Oils:

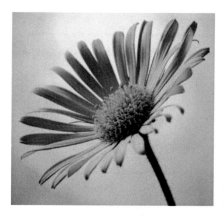

Arnica (*Arnica montana*) flowers are used in the maceration process, while the roots of the plant are used for homeopathic remedies. Arnica oil is useful as a compress, when used as soon as possible, on injuries with unbroken skin. Arnica oil is one of my favorites to reduce pain and inflammation for fractures, sprains, bruises, strained muscles, tendons, contusions, and swellings. In massage oil it is excellent to reduce muscle and joint inflammation.

Precautions: Arnica oil should only be used externally, not internally. Do not use on cuts or open wounds. It is best not to use arnica during pregnancy or while nursing. If taking blood-thinning medication, consult a physician.

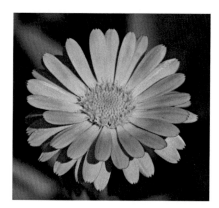

Calendula (*Calendula officinalis*) has incredible anti-inflammatory and vulnerary properties; it is found to be particularly useful for imbalances of the circulatory system. Its anti-inflammatory properties make it useful in balms and salves for wounds, bruises, bedsores, and skin rashes. The infused oil is excellent for skin care, particularly eczema. In addition, it is a perfect hydrosol to add to skin care products.

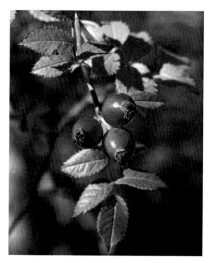

Rosehip (*Rosa canina*) is exceptional for tissue regeneration and for conditions such as facial wrinkles, premature aging, burns, and on scars following surgery. Rosehip's ability for skin regeneration and repair are due to high levels of both gamma-linolenic acid (47.4%) and linolenic fatty acids (33%).

These seeds also contain high levels of vitamin C, which assists the immune system and reduces the stress response.

Process of Oil Infusion

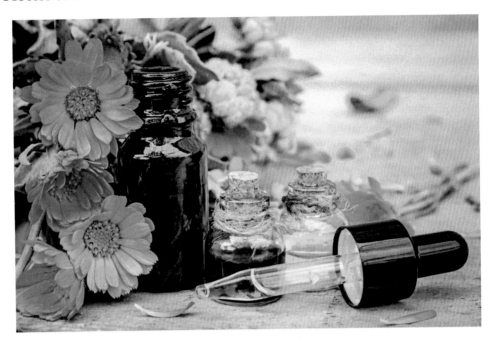

Oil Infusion:

STEP 1- Dry the flower heads, herbs, or plant material for a day or two.

Method- Dry plants by putting them in a basket with a cloth or paper towel in the bottom to soak up any moisture, hang them up, or place them in a paper bag.

STEP 2- Once the plant material is dry, you then chop, crush, or grind into small pieces or powder. You can infuse just one plant or a combination of plants like German chamomile (*Matricaria recutita*), rosehip (*Rosa canina*), and calendula (*Calendula officinalis*).

STEP 3- Place the plant material into a glass jar and cover with a base of either olive (*Olea europaea*) or jojoba (*Simmondsia chinensis*) oil. Both of these oils have a very long shelf life and will not go rancid. Jojoba (*Simmondsia chinensis*) is the best choice for delicate and more aromatic flowers. Remember to use a label with the ingredients and date of infusion.

STEP 4- This mixture is then left in a dark, warm environment for four to eight weeks, shaking the mixture daily 100 times, until the base oil has absorbed the properties and essential oils from the plant material. When you see the plant matter start to degrade it is time for the next step.

STEP 5- Drain off and filter the plant matter, using a funnel and strainer. Use an additional paper filter or cheese cloth if there are any small particles of plant matter.

STEP 6- Bottle - It is always best to store the finished product in a dark amber bottle.

STEP 7- Label- Include the common and botanical name of the plant and date of final processing and filtering.

Alcohol Infusion: With this process, you can use freshly harvested plant material and do not have to dry it first. This process is typically utilized for non-aromatic herb plants like Motherwort (*Leonurus cardiac*) and Echinacea Root (*Echinacea purpurea*) used as an herbal tincture. Follow the same instructions for the oil infusion.

Autumn Flower Essence

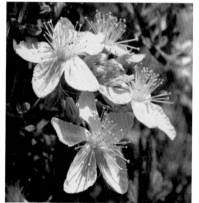

St. John's Wort (*Hypericum perforatum*)
"Hypericum" refers to its exalted status of solar brilliance at high summer. "Perforatum" is designated for the abundant oil glands which "perforate" the leaves and flowers of St. John's Wort, which allows the plants to hold light and warmth.

St. John's Wort flower essence has similar attributes as the whole herb, or tincture, with a few exceptions. As a flower essence, St. John's wort has impressive restorative powers, providing protection and strength when a person is overwhelmed or feeling physically or psychically vulnerable. This essence is useful for many levels of protection both psychically and environmentally and is suitable for those who are empathic.

Those that benefit from this flower essence may be sensitive to light and environmental factors, as well as feelings of anxiety and fear.

St. John's Wort flower essence is also useful for a wide variety of sleep disturbances such as insomnia, nightmares, night-sweats, and nighttime incontinence.

Encourages Positive Qualities:
Inner expansiveness
Radiance of spirit
Balanced renewal
"Radiant Protection"

Autumn Flower Essence

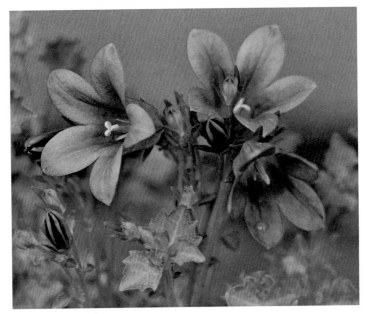

Creeping Bellflower
(*Campanula rapunculoides*)

Beneficial for highly sensitive people who feel troubled by hustle and bustle, stress, and noise, partly because they over-sympathize with others who are suffering.

Assists in opening the heart to self and others, and helps to clear negative beliefs.

Encourages Positive Qualities:
Calmness and centeredness
Integrated embodiment
"Conscious Integration"

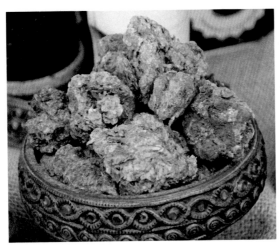

Autumn Hydrosol

Myrrh (*Commiphora myrrha*) has a resinous, woody-sweet aroma. The anti-microbial, anti-fungal, astringent and cicatrisant properties make this hydrosol very useful for supporting healthy skin, for wounds, cuts, or in skin care products, as well as in spritzers, facial toners, aftershave, mouth rinse or added into mouthwash.

Autumn Immune Strengthening

Living a healthy, natural life today can be an overwhelming challenge. We pack our schedules to the maximum; we often eat on the run, environmental toxins are everywhere; and stress levels are at an all-time high. All of these factors can impair our immune system. When the immune system is weak, the body becomes vulnerable, creating an opening for viruses and bacteria to invade. Maintaining a strong, healthy immune system is vital to achieving and retaining good health.

Strengthen your immune system naturally:

- Get adequate rest and sleep.
- Use essential oils regularly.
- Eat warm healthy foods.
- Eliminate processed and sugary foods.
- Reduce stress levels.
- Use herbal supplements: Omega 3 fatty acids, Vitamins B, C, and D.
- Exercise regularly.
- Meditate regularly.

Aromatherapy for Your Home and Office

Essential oils are natural immune system boosters. Their strong chemical components include anti-bacterial, antiviral, and antiseptic qualities.

Using aromatherapy in your home or office can quickly reduce stress, increase immunity, and create a pleasant ambiance.

Diffusing essential oils is one of the quickest ways to enhance immune stimulation and adds a wonderful ambiance to the environment. If you do not have a nebulizing diffuser you can also create a room spray or add a few drops of essential oils to a pot of hot water on the stove.

Autumn aromatherapy diffusing blends can bring comfort, warmth, and a burst of joy into your environment. These methods work quickly and do an excellent job of dispersing the essential oils throughout your home or office.

Aromatherapy Diffuser—Add twelve to twenty drops of a single essential oil or a blend into the nebulizing glass diffuser.

Autumn Diffuser Blends

The following aromatherapy blends are intended for use in a diffuser or in a room spritzer.

Radiant Uplifter Diffuser Blend

- **3 drops juniper** *(Juniperus communis)*
- **3 drops spruce** *(Picea mariana)*
- **3 drops gingergrass** *(Cymbopogon martinii var. sofia)*
- **3 drops spearmint** *(Mentha spicata)*

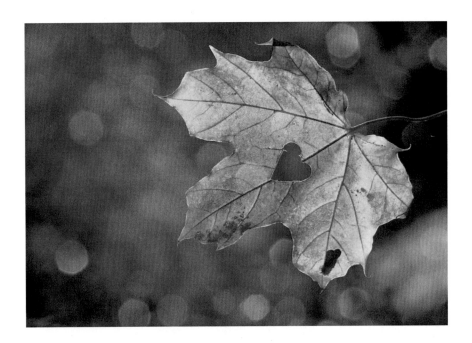

Chai Spice Diffuser Blend

- **6 drops cardamom** *(Elettaria cardamomum)*
- **3 drops clove** *(Syzygium aromaticum)*
- **3 drops ginger** *(Zingiber officinale)*
- **3 drops cinnamon** *(Cinnamomum verum)*

Nasal Inhaler: Aromatherapy's Unsung Hero

One of the unique features of aromatherapy, as an herbal healing modality, is the variety of applications. Of these, it is the aromatherapy inhalation application, the nasal inhaler, that is exceptionally effective, indeed aromatherapy's unsung hero. Here is why.

The sense of smell acts mostly on the subconscious level of the brain; yet it offers us more than 10,000 times more information than the senses of sight, taste, and touch combined.

The sense of smell (olfaction) was one of the earliest senses to arise in evolution, and it is well developed in animals. Olfaction is the process of the brain perceiving odor. It is utilized to detect odors of food, enemies, territory, and the opposite sex. In humans and animals, olfaction evokes emotional reactions that result in strong behavior changes.

When an essential oil is inhaled, the odor molecules travel up your nose where they are trapped by olfactory membranes. They are then carried to the limbic system where they pass between the major glands in the brain. From the limbic system, odor messages go to the hypothalamus, which sends messages to the other parts of the brain (pituitary, pineal, and amygdala) and body, stimulating the autonomic nervous system (ANS), endocrine system, organ functions, secretions of antibodies, neurotransmitters, hormones and enzymes throughout the body. The limbic system is where our memories, instincts, and vital functions are controlled and processed.

Smell is the only sense that goes directly to the limbic system, bypassing the cerebral cortex (our intellectual part of the brain). The other senses of sight and hearing must register with the cortex before entering other parts of the brain.

Many bodily functions, such as; digestive activity, respiration, hormone balance, heart rate, blood pressure, stress levels, pain reduction, and memory, can be regulated through the connection between the limbic system and other parts of the brain and body.

The effect of essential oils on the mind and emotions is extraordinary: uplifting depression, transforming anxiety into clarity, and stress into tranquility. Essential oils like sweet orange *(Citrus sinensis)* are known to be sedative while others are stimulating like rosemary *(Rosmarinus officinalis),* addressing the autonomic nervous system to produce the desired effect.

Odor messages are one of the fastest ways to achieve beneficial psychological or physiological effects. This extraordinary effect can take place in as little as ten seconds after inhaling an essential oil!

The olfactory system is the only sensory system that involves the amygdala and the limbic system in its primary processing pathway. This link explains why fragrances are often linked to specific memories. For example, if you have had a positive experience eating oranges as a child, then the aroma of sweet orange *(Citrus sinensis)* essential oil may also induce positive thoughts as an adult.

As stated in a Yale Scientific article, "Say for instance, when you inhale sweet orange *(Citrus sinensis)* essential oil, some of the minute molecules dissolve in the mucus lining of the olfactory epithelium on the roof of the nasal cavity. There, the molecules stimulate olfactory receptors. Olfactory sensory neurons carry the signals from the receptors to the olfactory bulb, which filters and begins processing the input signals of the orange fragrance. Mitral cells then carry the output signals from the olfactory bulb to the olfactory cortex, which allows you to perceive and recognize the tangy fragrance of the sweet orange *(Citrus sinensis)* essential oil.

Interestingly, the mitral cells do not only lead to the olfactory cortex, but they also carry the signals from the orange scent to other areas in the brain's limbic system. Some mitral cells connect directly to the amygdala, the brain structure involved in emotional learning and memory."[2]

The direct effect that odor can have on the hypothalamus, perhaps, suggests why aromatherapy is considered one of the most valuable tools in the treatment of stress and anxiety related conditions, which can be experienced as an overload of the sympathetic nervous system.

An *aromatherapy nasal inhaler* is an easy tool to engage your brain and nervous system responses and to stimulate your neurotransmitters. "Inhalation of essential oils can communicate signals to the olfactory system and stimulate the brain to exert neurotransmitters (e.g., serotonin and dopamine) thereby further regulating mood."[3]

The use of aromatherapy nasal inhalers is a much more concentrated inhalation application than just putting a drop of essential oil on a cotton ball, tissue, or even in a room diffuser. They are so easy and convenient to have on your desk, in your purse, backpack, pocket, or by your bedside table.

Since the essential oils are in the protective shell of the nasal inhaler tube, there is very little evaporation of the essential oils, and they have a very long shelf life. I have used nasal inhalers that are still potent for six months or longer.

The use of nasal inhalers has fewer precautions and safety issues to consider than other forms of aromatherapy applications, such as topical applications.

There are several parts to a nasal inhaler; the cover, insert, base cap, and a felt wick. If the felt wick is wrapped in a plastic coating, you may choose to substitute this for a cotton pad. If you are using a cotton pad, you may need to increase the number of essential oil drops.

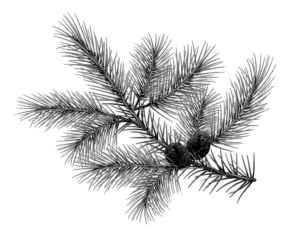

"Tree" essential oils and hydrosols are terrific for opening the respiratory system this time of year. The limbs of the trees are similar in structure to the bronchioles of the respiratory system.

These can be used in essential oil applications for strengthening the respiratory and digestive systems, by diffusing, in a nasal inhaler, aroma patch, room or shower spritzer, massage, or a topical blend.

Here are some of my favorite conifer essential oils to use during this time of year.

Fir, Silver (*Abies alba*) connects the body and mind, grounding, soothing. Increases and tonifies the lung energy. Used to reduce sinus issues, clear lung congestion, allergies, colds and flu.

Precautions: Old or oxidized oil should be avoided as it may cause skin sensitization if oxidized. May cause skin irritation in the bath.

Spruce, Black (*Picea mariana*) is a fantastic expectorant and ideal for many respiratory issues. It is a perfect remedy for many lung ailments such as asthma and bronchitis, especially when used in an inhalation blend. Black spruce essential oil is also known to support the adrenal glands during times of stress and fatigue. This oil is calming, grounding and creates a centering effect on the emotions.

Precautions: Oxidized oil should be avoided and may cause skin irritation in the bath.

Cypress *(Cupressus sempervirens)* is used in times of transition, such as; during career changes, moving, ending a close relationship, and times of significant spiritual changes or decisions. By nature, it is very grounding and cleansing. Cypress has an affinity for strengthening overburdened systems and restores calm. Also, it clears congestion in the respiratory system during the typical stresses of autumn and winter.

Precautions: Non-toxic, non-irritant when used in moderation.

Nasal inhaler Blend: Saturate the felt wick of a nasal inhaler with this blend of essential oils:

- **5 drops fir** *(Abies alba)*
- **5 drops cypress** *(Cupressus sempervirens)*
- **5 drops spruce** *(Picea mariana)*

Application: Inhale as needed to keep sinuses clear. Alternatively, for an Aroma Patch use one to two drops of each of the essential oils and apply underneath the clavicle.

Room or Shower Spritzer: In a 2oz. glass spray bottle, mix 15 drops of an essential oil blend into 1 tsp. of jojoba *(Simmondsia chinensis)*, or Solubol, shake well, and then add the liquid component of water and/or hydrosol.

Suggested blend for a shower spritzer:

> **5 drops of each:**
> - **fir** *(Abies alba)*
> - **spruce** *(Picea mariana)*
> - **manuka** *(Leptospermum scoparium)*

Application: Spray liberally into the upper corners of the shower before turning on the hot water.

Autumn is a dry season and one of the best times to stimulate the skin, circulatory, and lymphatic systems.

Dead Sea Salt Shower Scrub
Shower scrubs are fabulous to reduce dry skin, increase circulation and lymphatic flow, and to reduce pain and inflammation.

Makes about 1 cup / 8oz.

- Mix a combination of ½ cup each: fine grain **Dead Sea salt and sea salt.**
- Mix in 3-4 tablespoons of organic and **unrefined safflower** (*Carthamus tinctorius*) or **sesame** (*Sesamum indicum*) **oil.**

Mix in the essential oil blend:

- **8 drops fir** (*Abies alba*)
- **6 drops cypress** (*Cupressus sempervirens*)
- **6 drops spruce** (*Picea mariana*)

Apply the Dead Sea shower salt scrub two to three times a week, in the shower, before you turn the water on. Massage a small amount at a time with long smooth movements along the natural lymphatic flow, towards the heart (subclavian vein).

Salt Scrub Precautions- DO NOT apply the salt scrub to newly shaved areas, wounds, face, or breast tissue. Shower scrubs are not recommended for children. It is advised to review any precautions when using essential oils.

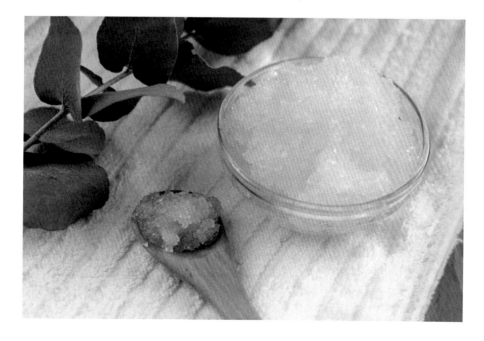

As the weather turns drier and colder you may feel your skin drying out. It's time for some nourishing healing salve, which has been a go-to product for me for many, many years.

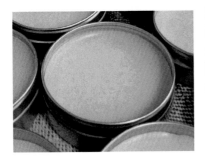

I want to share my favorite Healing Salve formulation with you. This salve is excellent for dry, irritated, and chapped skin, cuticles, dry heels, wounds, cuts, rashes, eczema, psoriasis, and even diaper rash.

Healing Salve - Makes 4oz.
Ingredients:

- **5 tablespoons grated unprocessed beeswax**
- **½ cup combination of carrier oils** (The last batch I made included a blend of **argan** (*Argania spinosa*), **calendula** (*Calendula officinalis*), **jojoba** (*Simmondsia chinensis*), **tamanu** (*Calophyllum inophyllum*), **wheat germ** (*Triticum vulgare*), and **Vitamin E.**)

Add the essential oils of your choice. 2% dilution in 4oz. (equals 48 drops). Try my favorite combination for deep skin nourishing:

- **15 drops helichrysum** (*Helichrysum italicum*)
- **15 drops lavender** (*Lavandula angustifolia*)
- **10 drops manuka** (*Leptospermum scoparium*)
- **8 drops calendula CO^2** (*Calendula officinalis*)

The dilution of essential oils will differ if using on a child. For small children, ages one to five, use .05%- six to ten drops per 4oz.

A suggested blend of essential oils for children:
3 to 5 drops **lavender** (*Lavandula angustifolia*)
3 to 5 drops **neroli** (*Citrus aurantium var. amara*)

Slowly melt beeswax in a double boiler. When the beeswax is melted, add in the carrier oils and stir well. Take off the heat, and just before a fine skin of wax forms, add the essential oils. Pour into glass jars and label. Refrigerate any extra you make to extend the shelf life.

Reminder: A small amount of healing salve goes a long way. A dime-sized amount is plenty to cover your cuticles or your heels.

Autumn Holistic Therapies

Lymphatic Drainage- if you tend to get sick during the Autumn this is a light touch therapy that strengthens the body's immune system and helps fight infection.

Massage- as mentioned previously, this healing modality is excellent any time of year. You might try a different technique like Thai massage or Rolfing to strengthen your structure.

Acupressure and Acupuncture- modalities that restore your vitality and strengthen your immune system in the Autumn. I am a bit needle shy, but the thin needles used in acupuncture are so worth the amazing results.

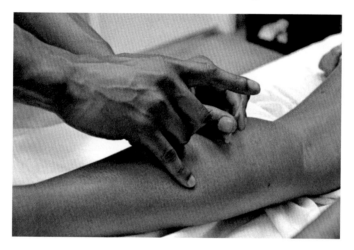

Self-Administered Modalities:

Self-Massage- once you get to know your anatomy, it is easy to work your hands, feet, legs, abdomen, and lower back. I often work on myself relieving small aches and pains before they become chronic. Self-massage is a wonderful way to care for your sacred body.

Tapping- useful to reduce emotional stress and rebalancing.

Autumn Quote

"Climb the mountains and get their good tidings. Nature's peace will flow into you as sunshine flows into trees. The winds will blow their own freshness into you, and the storms their energy, while cares will drop away from you like the leaves of Autumn."
John Muir, *The Mountains of California*

Chapter 6

Winter

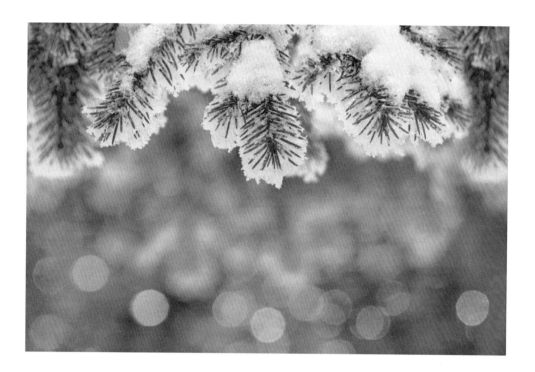

Winter is the perfect time for inward reflection, rest, recharge, and restoration. This season corresponds to the direction North; the darkest direction, to midnight, and the energy is cold, dark, and still. When we become still, we obtain a deeper awareness of ourselves without distortion. Winter is a good time for self-reflection and meditation, from which wisdom can emerge. When we become still and go within, we can reflect upon our life and prepare for new growth ahead in the springtime.

Body Care Tips for the Winter Season:

• **Take Time to Replenish:** Listen to your body and take time to replenish your reserves. Winter is a time to recharge and take time to go within. Get plenty of rest time and sleep.

• **Nourish Yourself:** Nourish yourself with warm food and beverages. Drink plenty of room temperature or warm water, no iced beverages. Eat warming foods such as root vegetables, whole grains, and small amounts of meat or fish protein. If you are a vegetarian eat more beans, nuts, and tempeh. Add extra oil to your diet like flaxseed oil or avocados.

• **Keep Warm:** Prepare for the weather and dress accordingly. Keep yourself well covered when out of doors. The neck, shoulders, abdomen, and on the back around the kidneys are more sensitive to cold and wind.

The element of water is connected to this time of year. Water is the key component to life and continued growth. Staying hydrated is crucial; our body weight is 60% water. As we age we lose water, and our bodies begin to dry out. This can be reflected in our bones and hair, which become more brittle, and our skin loses its youthful elasticity.

If you experience headaches, muscle cramps, reduced sweating, reduced urination, constipation, or overheating you could be dehydrated. Women generally need, on average, nine cups (or more during nursing), of water a day, and men need up to thirteen cups a day. There are variations to these amounts depending on the climate and altitude where you live and your daily activity.

Other physical challenges that can occur if this element is weak:

- Lower back pain, chronic or acute.
- Knee pain and weakness.
- Bone, teeth, and hearing issues.
- Problems with urinary retention.
- Vertigo or dizziness.
- Sexual problems that can include lack of excitement, premature ejaculation, and vaginal dryness.
- Weakness of vitality.

Winter Emotion

Fear is the emotion associated with the winter season. Healthily, fear is an emotion that moves and directs us to remain alert and attentive to our surroundings and situation. When confronted with danger, constructive fear can guide us with a message of caution and restraint and fill us with a sense of readiness and courage to face whatever situation life might present.

Fortunately, this season encourages the ability to listen deeply within ourselves. When we are healthy we engage in a robust response to life, neither by running away (excess fear) nor by reckless attacking (lack of fear).

The beneficial energy of this season can generate persistence, will, and diligence to go through the darkest and most challenging of times.

> *"If you look into your own heart, and you find nothing wrong there, what is there to worry about? What is there to fear?" Confucius*

Winter Herbs- Used in tea, capsules, and tinctures:

At the first signs of immune system weakness, use these effective herbals. The adult dosage of tinctures is usually taken by the dropper full directly or added to water. A dropper equals approximately 30 drops.

Ashwagandha root *(Withania somnifera)* is known as an adaptogenic herb (improves your ability to respond to stress) and popular in Ayurvedic medicine. It has shown incredible results for reducing anxiety and stress, improving brain function, and hormonal support.

Astragalus root *(Astragalus propinquus)* a stimulant for the immune system. It is an antioxidant that inhibits free radical production. In the body, free radicals damage cells and are linked to many health problems associated with aging. I use it as a general tonic and to fight bacteria and viruses.

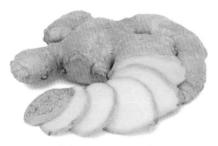

Ginger root *(Zingiber officinale)* is from the Zingiberaceae family and is one of the most commonly consumed dietary condiments in the world. Its spicy aroma is mainly due to the presence of ketones, especially the gingerols, which appear to be the primary chemical component of ginger. It is a savory addition for your winter meals or as a warming tea with honey.

Ginger has been used for thousands of years to reduce a variety of ailments, such as digestive issues, colds, nausea, arthritis, migraines, and hypertension. It can decrease inflammation, swelling, and pain.

Olive leaf (*Olea europaea*) an excellent immune support. Olive leaves contain high amounts of oleuropein, a polyphenol with unique health-improving attributes. This herb has been used in traditional medicine for centuries to improve age-related diseases. The oleuropein in olive leaf is a natural wide-spectrum antibiotic, antibacterial, antiviral, and antifungal.

Another product I have on hand during the winter months, to use as needed, is Colloidal Silver. It is worth mentioning, even though it is not from an herb, as it is very useful as an anti-microbial, immune stimulant and is safe for children and during pregnancy. I use this product as well as other herbs, tinctures, and herbal capsules instead of traditional antibiotics. There are many brands of colloidal silver, but I am partial to using Silvercillin™ from Designs for Health.

Winter Flower Essence

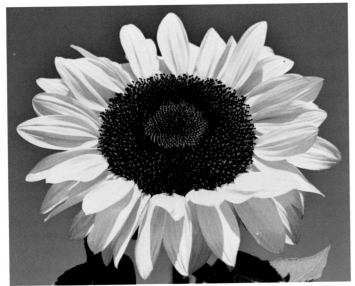

Sunflower
(*Helianthus annuus*)
Sunflower radiates the sun energies. When this plant is growing the blossom follows the sun.

Used as a flower essence, it is a remedy to uplift one's spirits and create a personal glow from the inside out. Sunflower is an energizer that can banish any feelings of the doldrums. It gives one the courage to show one's true self to others. Sunflower is an excellent confidence builder for use anytime you are feeling nervous about doing something.

Encourages Positive Qualities:
Optimism and Self-esteem
Warmth and radiance of spirit
"Positivity in Adversity"

Winter Hydrosol

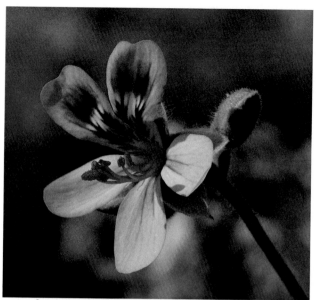

Geranium, Rose
(Pelargonium graveolens var. roseum)
Rose geranium hydrosol has a rosy floral aroma. It has a balancing effect on the nervous system, uplifting the spirit and a balancing effect on the adrenal cortex and the hormonal system.

It is a mild astringent with antibacterial properties. It is useful for acne, dermatitis, eczema, and oily complexions. It assists in balancing the secretion of sebum and clears sluggish and oily skin. It is also a helpful aid to assist with burns, wounds, ulcers, and other skin problems.

Moderately stable shelf life: 12 to14 months, best to keep refrigerated.

Wintertime is All About the Bath

Winter is the perfect time for an aromatherapy bath to restore, integrate, replenish, and relax. Adding essential oils into a bath is a fast and effective way to use aromatherapy and to derive immeasurable healing benefits.

There are several effective ways to add essential oils into a bathtub. One is to add five to twelve drops of essential oils into one tablespoon of jojoba oil *(Simmondsia chinensis)*, castile soap or Solubol. Mix the ingredients, and then add to the running bath water. Using the jojoba oil *(Simmondsia chinensis)*, castile soap, or Solubol assists the essential oils to disperse into the bath water, not adhere onto the walls of the bathtub. If you are using Solubol, it is blended at a ratio of one to four, i.e. to every drop of essential oil, add four drops Solubol.

Add your chosen emulsifier to the following aromatherapy bath blends:

Favorite essential oil blend for stimulating morning wake-up:

- **4 drops rose geranium** *(Pelargonium roseum)*
- **2 drops palmarosa** *(Cymbopogon martinii)*
- **2 drops jasmine** *(Jasminum grandiflorum)*

Favorite essential oil blend for soothing evening relaxation:

- **4 drops Roman chamomile** *(Anthemis nobilis)*
- **2 drops ylang ylang** *(Cananga odorata)*
- **2 drops vetiver** *(Vetiveria zizanoides)*

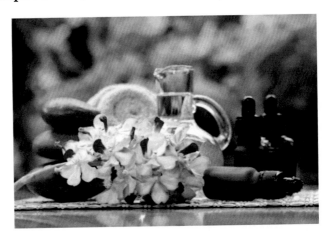

Favorite to strengthen and restore overburdened systems; calms nervous tension and stress related conditions:

- **4 drops cardamom** *(Elettaria cardamomum)*
- **3 drops rhododendron** *(Rhododendron anthopogon)*
- **3 drops vetiver** *(Vetiveria zizanoides)*

Favorite essential oil blend for soothing skin:

- **4 drops lavender** *(Lavandula angustifolia)*
- **2 drops petitgrain** *(Citrus aurantium)*
- **2 drops rose** *(Rosa damascena)*

These blends can be used in the bath, shower salt scrub, or just the essential oil blend, without a carrier oil, can be used in a diffuser or nasal inhaler.

Use a 0.5-1% dilution (three to six drops total) for children under seven, during pregnancy and nursing, for elders, or those with sensitive skin.

Essential Oil Bath Precautions

Choosing essential oils for your bath does require some thought as to the precautions. Please DO NOT add essential oils that are skin irritants into a bath such as, citrus oils, or the spice oils like; cinnamon *(Cinnamomum zeylanicum)*, thyme *(Thymus vulgaris)*, oregano *(Origanum vulgare)*, peppermint *(Mentha x piperita)*, ginger *(Zingiber officinale)* and black pepper *(Piper nigrum)*, or essential oils that are old and can be oxidized.

Essential Oil Bath Dilutions

- Children, under one year, should have no more than one drop of essential oil per bath. Salt and clay baths are not recommended.
- Children, between one and four, as well as for pregnant women, add only two drops of essential oil per bath.
- Children, between the ages of four and twelve, as well as for elderly people, just add two to four drops of essential oil per bath.
- Adults, add five-ten drops of essential oil per bath.

Adding salt to your bathing routine is an easy and powerful way to boost your circulation, reduce general fatigue and inflammation, and to cleanse your energy body.

Salt Baths

Sea salt, Dead Sea salt, or Epsom salts.

Start by adding two to four cups of salt into the running bath water.

Then, mix five to ten drops of essential oils into one tablespoon of jojoba oil *(Simmondsia chinensis)*, castile soap, or Solubol and add this to the running bath water.

Favorite essential oil blend to reduce inflammation~

Mix your chosen emulsifier into the following essential oil blend.

- **4 drops helichrysum** *(Helichrysum italicum)*
- **2 drops neroli** *(Citrus aurantium)*
- **2 drops cypress** *(Cupressus sempervirens)*

Shower Salt Scrub

Makes 4oz. Combine the following ingredients:

- **½ cup of salt** (Combination of fine grain Dead Sea Salt and sea salt.)
- **2-3 tablespoons of organic safflower** (*Carthamus tinctorius*) oil

    Essential oil blend:

- **5 drops lemongrass** (*Cymbopogon citratus*)
- **4 drops black pepper** (*Piper nigrum*)
- **3 drops ginger** (*Zingiber officinale*)

Apply two to three times a week in a dry shower, before you turn the water on. Massage a small amount at a time with long smooth movements along the natural lymphatic flow, toward the heart. Since salt absorbs, it is best to store it in a glass container if it will not be used immediately.

Precautions: This blend is *not* recommended to use in the bath, because the essential oils are all skin irritants. Not for children under age fourteen. DO NOT apply to newly shaved areas, on the face, cuts, wounds, or the breast tissue.

If you still feel aches and pains after a shower or bath you can use this topical aromatherapy blend:

Topical Pain Relief Blend

Makes 1 oz. Combine the following ingredients:

- **1 oz. arnica infused oil** (*Arnica montana*)
- **5 drops lemongrass** (*Cymbopogon citratus*)
- **4 drops black pepper** (*Piper nigrum*)
- **3 drops ginger** (*Zingiber officinale*)

Precautions: DO NOT apply on wounds or cuts. Not for use in the bath. Not for use with children.

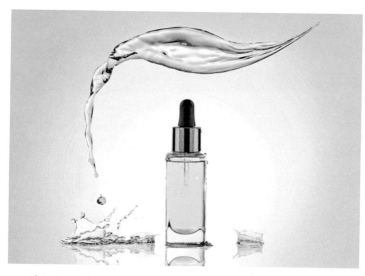

**Carrier Oils
for Winter**

Winter is the most challenging season to keep the skin supple and nourished.

Natural skin care can nourish, soothe, and correct any imbalance in the skin's ph.

Look radiant, youthful and enjoy a natural, healthy glow, even during the darkest, driest months of the year.

Carrier, or base oils, are the fats extracted from seeds, nuts, grains, vegetables, and fruits, and they are used as a base for various skin care products. Many vegetable oils, such as olive *(Olea europaea)* and jojoba *(Simmondsia chinensis)*, are already popular for both cosmetic and medicinal purposes. For best results always choose carrier oils that are unrefined, cold pressed, organic, and unfractionated.

There are many wonderful carrier oils that you can use for facial serums. Here are a few of my favorites.

Argan *(Argania spinosa)*
Common Uses: Excellent for moisturizing, conditioning, and healing the skin. Used for a facial serum, massage oil, hair serum, hand and cuticle repair, soothes dry elbows and heels.
Shelf Life: Two years, if refrigerated after opening.

Camellia seed *(Camellia sinensis)*
Common Uses: Camellia oil protects the skin from free radical damage, refines mature skin, and nourishes the complexion. It is easily absorbed by the skin, leaving it silky smooth without the greasy feeling, making it one of the best-kept secrets in the cosmetic and hair care industry. For centuries, it has been used as a traditional hair conditioner and also as a treatment to strengthen brittle nails.
Shelf Life: Two years, if refrigerated after opening.

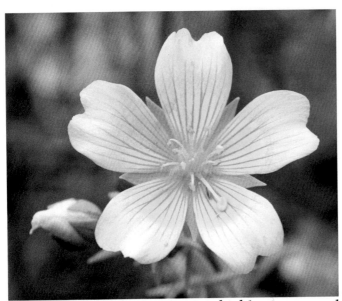

Meadowfoam
(Limnanthes alba) is resistant to oxidation due to naturally occurring tocopherols and is one of the most stable lipids known. It will extend the shelf life of less stable ingredients. As a result, it has an extremely long shelf life.
Common Uses: Meadowfoam has wonderful moisturizing and rejuvenating properties. It is highly recommended for use in cosmetics and skin care products, especially for its UV protection properties.

It is a key ingredient in many different products, such as; suntan lotion, massage oils, lotions, hand/facial creams, hair and scalp products, cuticle repair cream, foundations, lip balms, shampoos, shaving creams, and balms.
Shelf Life: Two years, if refrigerated after opening.

Red raspberry *(Rubus idaeus)*
Common Uses: This nourishing and healing oil is an excellent choice for use in healing salves, serums, and other skin care formulations. It has exceptional anti-inflammatory properties that make it one of the best carrier oils for assisting eczema, psoriasis and other skin conditions.
Shelf Life: One to two years, if refrigerated after opening.

Aromatherapy Facial Serum is healing, nourishing, toning, and regenerating to the skin surface and individual skin cells. The carrier oils and essential oils have properties proven to improve skin tone and elasticity for mature or dry skin. They also stimulate the production of new cells which can deter and slow wrinkles.

Enjoy one of my favorite facial serum formulations:
In a 2-oz. amber glass bottle, with a pump top, mix:

- **1 tablespoon argan** (*Argania spinosa*)
- **1/2 tablespoon camellia seed** (*Camellia sinensis*)
- **1/2 tablespoon red raspberry** (*Rubus idaeus*)
- **1/4 tablespoon meadowfoam** (*Limnanthes alba*)
- **1/4 tablespoon borage** (*Borago officinalis*)
- **1 teaspoon jojoba** (*Simmondsia chinensis*)

Then add, the following essential oils:

- **6 drops rose** (*Rosa damascena*)
- **5 drops neroli** (*Citrus aurantium*)
- **3 drops vetiver** (*Vetiveria zizanoides*)
- **3 drops petitgrain** (*Citrus aurantium*)

Shake well and apply two to four drops after cleansing the face and using an aromatherapy facial spritzer. *Precaution: During pregnancy reduce the dilution of essential oils to ½ to 1%.

This facial serum can also be applied as an oil face wash.

Do not be afraid of applying oil to your face. Oil, alone, will not contribute to blemishes, which are generally a result of several different factors, including hormones, bacteria, dead skin cells, and the buildup of these factors. Your skin naturally produces oil because it requires it.

The natural oils assist in protecting and lubricating the skin so that it may function naturally. Properly functioning skin is beautiful, radiant, and glowing.

Oil Face Wash Application:

Make sure you have your aromatherapy facial oil blend, a soft washcloth, and hot water.

- Squirt ½-1 tablespoon of the aromatherapy facial oil blend into the palm of your hand.
- Gently cover your face with the oil blend.
- Massage this blend into your face and neck for three to five minutes. This will remove sunscreen, makeup, dirt, and other impurities. There is no need to use a makeup remover or to wash your face with soap before the massage.
- Take your time... This is an excellent opportunity for deep breathing, relaxing and releasing some of your stress.
- Next, soak your washcloth in clean, warm water. The water needs to be warm enough to soften your pores and remove the oil.
- Hold the washcloth to cover your face. Keep it on your face until it starts to cool down. You will feel your pores softening and releasing the impurities. Gently
wipe the oil away and rinse the washcloth well in hot, running water.
- Wipe gently, rinse thoroughly, and then repeat two or three more times. It is important not to scrub your face, wipe gently. Let the oil and warm water do the work for you.

Body Butter is another product that I have on hand for nourishing winter skin. Enjoy one of my favorite body butter formulations.

Makes 8 oz.

Ingredients:

- **1 cup raw shea butter** *(Vitellaria paradoxa)* OR coconut oil *(Cocos nucifera)*
- **4 tablespoon grated yellow beeswax** *(Apis mellifica)*
- **4 tablespoon carrot seed oil** *(Daucus carota)*
- **4 tablespoon red raspberry seed oil** *(Rubus idaeus)*
- **4 tablespoon wheat germ oil** *(Triticum vulgare)*
- **2 tablespoon macadamia oil** *(Macadamia integrifolia)*
- **2 tablespoon jojoba oil** *(Simmondsia chinensis)*
- **½ tablespoon vitamin E**, 5,000 IU (a-tocopherol)

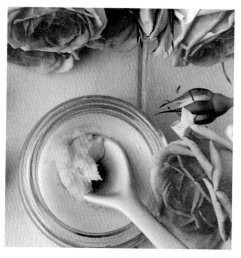

Add the essential oils:

10 drops rose
(Rosa centifolia)

10 drops lavender
(Lavandula angustifolia)

15 drops palmarosa
(Cymbopogon martinii)

Use a lower dilution (1%) of the essential oils for children: no more than six drops per ounce.

This final product is thick. Use less beeswax to formulate a more liquid product.

Directions:

1. In a double boiler, over low heat, melt the shea butter OR coconut oil, and beeswax. Once these ingredients are melted, add the other carrier oils, getting them all to the same temperature.
2. Remove from heat and allow slight cooling prior to adding the essential oils.
3. Pour into a glass jar or BPA-free plastic bottle with a flip top.
4. Allow to cool at room temperature. Seal the containers and label.

Shelf life is for 30 days, when stored in a cool cupboard. Refrigerate to extend shelf life.

Winter Holistic Therapies

Winter is the perfect time for Hot Stone Massage which melts away tension, eases muscle stiffness, and increases circulation. It can also reduce muscle spasms and improve flexibility and range of motion.

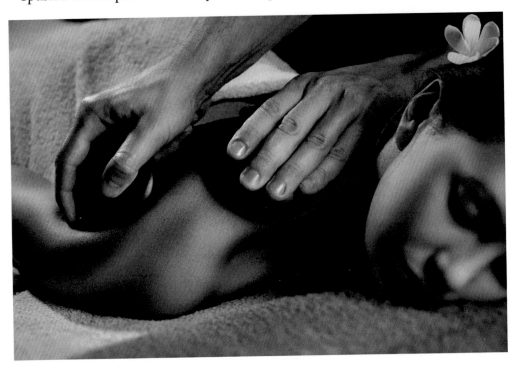

Winter Quote

"Winter is the time for comfort, for good food and warmth, for the touch of a friendly hand and for a talk beside the fire: it is the time for home."
Edith Sitwell

Chapter 7

Spring

Springtime symbolizes the beginning stages of new life and creation. It is expansive, moving out in all directions. This season corresponds to the direction of the East; dawn, when the buds come out on the trees and turn into young green leaves, when seeds that have lain dormant under the earth all winter push up through the ground as sprouts.

Warmth and light begin to return; the soil is moist with the winter melt, and the days are now longer than the nights. The wood phase also corresponds to the seeds that have lain dormant in the earth all winter. They grow, push up through the ground as tender sprouts, then buds develop and turn into young green leaves. It is the time when we are once again moved to spend more time outdoors in the freshness of a spring morning.

Springtime energy provides us with the sense of renewal, reawakening, and rebirth. It gives us a connection to the future, which allows us to plan and design in all areas of our lives, giving us the ability to initiate thoughts, plans, and activities. It helps us to coordinate our ideas and feelings, bringing them into action and change. This energy provides us with vision and foresight to move ahead, even when we are challenged with obstacles, allowing us to express our true nature, and to manifest this creative energy into the world. Other attributes of this season are considered to be strength and flexibility, like bamboo.

Spring Cleaning

Spring is the time to open the windows, clean out the closets and clean your home environment. Using essential oils in household cleaning is the safest and healthiest way to enhance your health and the environment. Commercial cleansers contain ingredients that are toxic and pose many health hazards.

Some commercial cleaners can cause acute or immediate hazards, such as skin or respiratory irritation, watery eyes, or chemical burns; while others are associated with chronic, or long-term illness. We use a wide array of scents, soaps, detergents, bleaching agents, softeners, scourers, polishes, and specialized cleaners for bathrooms, glass, drains, and ovens to keep our homes sparkling and sweet-smelling. These chemicals, which are in cleaning foams, bleach, and disinfectant work to make our dishes, bathtubs, and countertops gleaming and germ-free, but many also contribute to indoor air pollution, are poisonous if ingested, and can be harmful if inhaled or touched.

Fragrances, added to many cleaners, most notably laundry detergents and fabric softeners, may cause acute effects such as; respiratory irritation, headache, sneezing, and watery eyes in sensitive individuals or allergy and asthma sufferers.

The National Institute of Occupational Safety and Health has found that one-third of the substances used in the fragrance industry are toxic. Because the chemical formulas of fragrances are considered trade secrets, companies aren't required to list their ingredients but merely label them as containing "fragrance." * Please note that "fragrances" are NOT true essential oils.

Other ingredients in cleaners may have low acute toxicity but contribute to long-term health effects, such as cancer or hormone disruption. Many commercial all-purpose cleaners contain the sudsing agents diethanolamine (DEA) and triethanolamine (TEA). When these substances come into contact with nitrites, often present as undisclosed preservatives or contaminants, they react to form nitrosamines - carcinogens that readily penetrate the skin. 1,4-dioxane, another suspected carcinogen, may be present in cleaners made with ethoxylated alcohols. Butyl cellosolve (also known as ethylene glycol monobutyl ether), which may be neurotoxic (or cause damage to the brain and nervous system),
is also present in some cleaners.

The good news is that there are simple and effective natural ingredients for cleaning.

Essential oils can be added to castile soap, water, baking soda, white vinegar, and lemon juice, which can take care of most household cleaning needs.

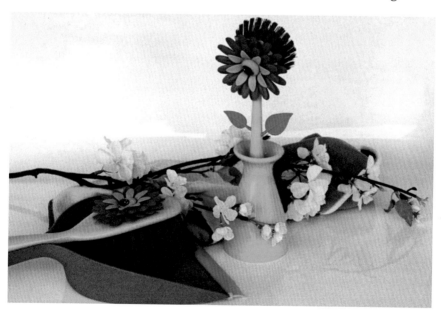

A few of my favorite essential oils for cleaning are Lemon (*Citrus limon*), Peppermint (*Mentha piperita*), Eucalyptus (*Eucalyptus radiata* or *Eucalyptus citriodora*), and Cedarwood (*Cedrus atlantica*).

Aromatherapy Household Cleaning

Add essential oils to your spring-cleaning.

Damp Mop- add two to three drops of a favorite essential oil to a wet mop.

Lemon *(Citrus limon)* a powerful anti-bacterial, antioxidant, anti-viral, and immune stimulant.

Eucalyptus *(Eucalyptus radiata)* useful anti-viral, anti-bacterial, anti-fungal, anti-infectious, antiseptic, deodorant, and insecticidal.

Carpets- add two to four drops of essential oil to ½ cup of baking soda and sprinkle on carpets before vacuuming.

Peppermint *(Mentha piperita)* useful anti-fungal, anti-parasitic, antibacterial, anti-viral, and respiratory support.

Eucalyptus *(Eucalyptus radiata)* useful anti-viral, anti-bacterial, anti-fungal, anti-infectious, antiseptic, deodorant, and insecticidal.

Furniture Dusting- add two to four drops of essential oil to a soft, damp cloth.

Lemon *(Citrus limon)* a powerful anti-bacterial, antioxidant, anti-viral, and immune stimulant.

Closets- packing away your winter clothes? Instead of using something like mothballs, apply one to three drops of cedarwood *(Cedrus atlantica)* essential oil on a cotton ball.

Cedarwood *(Cedrus atlantica)* effective anti-fungal, antibacterial, antiseptic, astringent, and an insect repellent.

Diffusing- After a good house cleaning, diffusing or a room spritzer will enhance and cleanse the environment.

Citrus Room Spritzer

In a 2oz. glass bottle, with a spray top, add the following ingredients:

- **1 teaspoon jojoba** *(Simmondsia chinensis)* or Solubol.

  Add the essential oils and remaining liquid:

  - **6 drops orange** *(Citrus sinensis)*
  - **8 drops grapefruit** *(Citrus x paradisi)*
  - **4 drops lemon** *(Citrus limon)*
  - **4 drops lime** *(Citrus aurantifolia)*
  - **1 oz. spearmint** *(Mentha spicata)* hydrosol and then purified water to fill the bottle.

First, put the jojoba *(Simmondsia chinensis)*, or Solubol into the bottom of the bottle, add the essential oils, and shake well. Then, add in the water and hydrosol. Shake well.

Spray in the corners of a room or on linens. Caution: Keep away from the face.

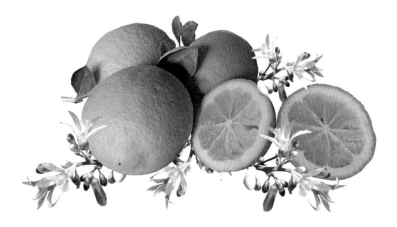

Springtime is also an optimum time to cleanse the body, particularly the liver and intestines. The liver is the largest solid organ in the body, located in the upper right abdomen. It is a vital internal organ for aiding digestion. The liver also filters the blood and removes waste products and worn-out cells from the blood. The liver also detoxifies chemicals and metabolizes drugs.

The liver converts food into substances needed for life and growth, storing glycogen (a blood-sugar regulator), amino acids, protein, and fat. It also makes the enzymes and bile that help to digest food. The liver neutralizes harmful toxins and wastes, so it is at high risk of contamination from environmental toxins, and those contained in over-processed foods. The liver has over 500 different functions; it is the body's chemical factory and the most significant blood cleansing internal organ.

Why Should You do an Internal Cleanse?

Cleansing the body rids excess waste and dis-ease. It rejuvenates the vital energy of physical, mental, and emotional well-being. Signs of internal toxicity can include; headaches, backaches, allergies, skin rashes, constipation, fatigue, immune weakness, insomnia, digestive issues, frequent colds, and general inflammation and weakness. With the proper cleansing and detoxification of the body we can maintain health and vitality, even as we age.

As Elson Haas, M.D., mentions in his book *The Detox Diet*, "We also cleanse/detoxify to rest or heal our overloaded digestive organs and allow them to catch up on past work. At the same time, we are inspired to cleanse our external life as well, cleaning out our rooms, sorting through the piles on our desks, and clarifying our personal priorities. Most often our energy is increased and becomes steadier, motivating us to change both internally and externally.

'Life's Great Law: Every living cell of the organized body is endowed with an instinct of self-preservation, sustained by an inherent force in the organism called 'vital force,' or 'life force.' Creating better health and a higher level of life force depends on the function of your body, mind, and emotions. The state of health is evident in your internal organs, blood and lymphatic system. The main internal organs to keep functioning optimally are your intestines, liver, and kidneys."[1]

For the last twenty-five years I have done an internal cleanse at least once a year. The duration of the cleanse varies depending on the congestion that I experience in my body and mind. Generally, if I feel healthy, then a three to five day cleanse is adequate. If I am suffering with more inflammation and have foggy thinking, then I cleanse ten to twenty-one days.

Note: Pregnancy is *not* a suitable time for cleansing the body.
It is also not recommended for children under 14. If you have an existing health condition, please consult with your health care provider.

Simple ways to start the daily cleansing process:

- Drink three to four glasses of water with one to two tablespoons lemon juice (not essential oil)

Include the following foods into your diet:

- Lots of green leafy vegetables in your diet: like kale, Swiss chard, dandelion, and spinach
- Avocados
- Green tea, instead of other caffeinated beverages
- Garlic
- Citrus fruit
- Vegetable juicing and smoothies

How to Begin an Internal Cleanse

If you are new to internal cleansing it is best to start the process slowly so that you do not detox too quickly. Here are simple ways to start the internal cleansing process, which can be a one-day to three-month process:

1) Reduce or eliminate congestive foods like meat, poultry, dairy, alcohol, caffeine, sugar, processed foods, and all nightshade vegetables (tomatoes, potatoes, peppers, and eggplant), which can increase inflammation.

2) Start your day with two to three, eight-ounce glasses of purified water with one to two teaspoons of lemon juice (the juice from the fruit, not the essential oil). Then, continue drinking filtered water with the lemon juice throughout the day.

3) Include the following foods into your diet to cleanse your liver:

- LOTS of green leafy vegetables like kale, Swiss chard, dandelion, and spinach.
- MORE vegetables.
- Avocados.
- Green tea.
- Garlic.
- Citrus fruits.
- Turmeric (*Curcuma longa*): As a ground spice or in capsules; reduces inflammation.
- Powdered greens: spirulina, chlorella, blue-green algae. Noted as the "super" foods.
- Vegetable juicing and smoothies: Fantastic way to get vital vitamins and nutrients into the body quickly.
- Digestive enzymes and probiotics: These quickly remove toxins out of the digestive system.

Spring Herbs

Herbs are fantastic cleansers for the liver and gall bladder.
The following herbs should be used in teas, decoctions, or tinctures:

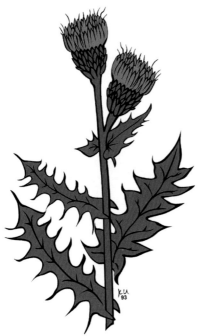

Milk Thistle (*Silybum marianum*) has been used for over two thousand years due to its remarkable effects on the liver and gallbladder. Galen and Pliny, the ancient philosophers, recognized and used the power of milk thistle for liver cleansing and support. This herb contains silymarin, which protects the liver from toxins, and helps with the detoxification of poisons such as alcohol. It can help to regenerate damaged liver tissue, stimulate bile production, and improve digestion.

Yellow Dock (*Rumex crispus*) known as a blood purifier and commonly used to cleanse toxins from the body. Yellow dock helps break down fatty foods by stimulating bile production, enhancing normal liver detoxification, improving the flow of digestive juices, helping the liver eliminate toxins, and it has mild diuretic effects to help flush out harmful substances. It also helps reduce irritation of the liver and digestive system.

Burdock root or seed (*Arctium lappa*) a liver cleansing agent. It is useful to reduce skin conditions, including eczema, psoriasis, and dermatitis. These conditions often manifest when the liver is overloaded from a diet high in fat and protein. Burdock aids the liver in metabolizing these nutrients and encourages the removal of waste products. This is one reason why burdock is considered a blood tonic.

Burdock also aids in the removal of uric acid waste products, which makes it useful for those who suffer from joint conditions such as gout, rheumatoid arthritis, and bursitis. Such conditions often result from an excess of acidic waste products. Both burdock root and seed can act as a diuretic, making it useful for people who experience swelling in the hands and feet. Burdock root is safe to use during pregnancy for this purpose, but the seed should be avoided during pregnancy.

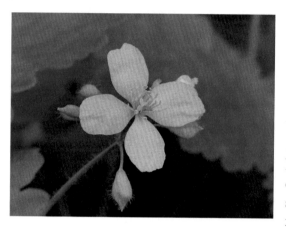

Celandine, Greater (*Chelidonium majus*) the ancient Greeks and Romans considered celandine to be one of the most powerful liver cleansing herbs. Maurice Mességué, a famous French herbalist, used greater celandine for all liver problems. Celandine helps to improve a sluggish liver eliminate foreign particles, stimulate the production of bile, relieve gallbladder spasms, and stimulate enzyme production from the pancreas.

Chanca Piedra (*Phyllanthus niruri*) has been used for centuries by indigenous people of the Amazon to promote the body's natural processes of the liver, gallbladder, and kidney. It also stimulates the liver to purge itself of harmful toxins and foreign particles. Chanca piedra soothes the liver, increases bile production, and reduces the formation of calcified stones in the body. "This herb is also known as, 'the stone breaker.' It is useful for digestive tract disorders including: gas, loss of appetite, stomachache, intestinal infections, constipation, and dysentery."[2]

Chicory root (*Cichorium intybus*) a medicinal herb celebrated for its ability to help cleanse the liver. Ancient Roman, Persian, Arabian, and Indian physicians used chicory leaves and root to aid against a slew of liver ailments including; jaundice, gallbladder and liver stones, urinary stones, constipation, indigestion, depression, and headaches.

Dandelion *(Taraxacum officinale)* many people think of the dandelion as a pesky weed; however, it is chock full of vitamins A, B, C, and D, as well as minerals, such as iron, potassium, and zinc. Dandelion leaves are used to add flavor to salads, sandwiches, and teas. The roots are used in some coffee substitutes, and the flowers are used to make wines. In the past, dandelion roots and leaves were used to treat liver problems. Native Americans also boiled dandelion in water and took it to treat kidney disease, swelling, skin problems, heartburn, and upset stomach.

Spring Flower Essence

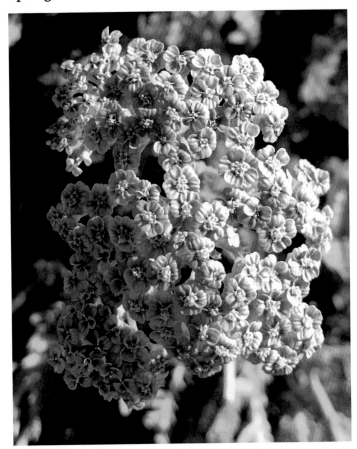

Occasionally, during a cleanse, you can feel out of sorts or irritable as things in your bodymind are balancing out.

Pink Yarrow (Achillea millefolium var. rosea) flower essence can be a soothing companion.

Pink Yarrow corresponds to the "root" chakra, the red chakra. It imparts a strong sense of grounded-ness.

Helpful for those who lack a good, confident sense of self and look to complete themselves in relation to other people. This can result in imbalanced relationships where they "give too much" and try to solve other people's problems so that they don't have to feel other people's pain.

Encourages Positive Qualities:
Sense of self-worth
Empathy, not sympathy
"Rooted Empathy"

Spring Hydrosols

Hydrosols are waters containing beneficial plant compounds, a result of extraction by distillation. 'Hydro' means water and 'sol' means solution. These hydrosols or herbal distillates have many uses as medicine, flavorings, household uses and as fabulous additions to skin care products. They are generally safer than essential oils to use with children, elders, and those with sensitive skin.

As I mentioned in Chapter 3, many hydrosols can also be used internally in moderation. Please see complete instructions in these book references:
Hydrosols: The Next Aromatherapy by Suzanne Catty
375 Essential Oils and Hydrosols by Jeanne Rose.

Carrot seed *(Daucus carota)* believed to cleanse and support the liver and gallbladder. Carrot seed hydrosol can detoxify the blood, tissues, muscles.

Helichrysum *(Helichrysum italicum)* a most potent anti-inflammatory. It is useful after surgery, healing of wounds, reducing swelling, and a detoxifier for the liver.

Labrador tea *(Ledum groenlandicum)*

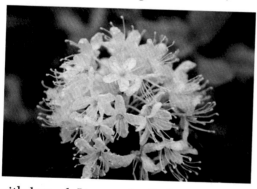

Suzanne Catty, in her book, describes "Labrador Tea Hydrosol as being the most powerfully therapeutic of all hydrosols."[3] Catty also describes Labrador Tea as being helpful for fighting addictive behaviors and suggests blending it with yarrow *(Achillea millefolium)* hydrosol to aid with withdrawal. It may also be helpful with allergies, liver, and kidney detoxification, and it is an immune stimulant.

Myrtle, Green *(Myrtus communis)* cleansing for the liver. This specific hydrosol also makes a good eyewash for tired, irritated eyes or allergic conjunctivitis. Green myrtle is a strong expectorant useful for bronchitis and allergies.

Yarrow *(Achillea millefolium)* a good digestive aid and is detoxifying. Regular use of this hydrosol during cleansing can improve digestion, elimination, and calm gastric spasms.

Spring Essential Oils

While doing an internal cleanse, essential oils are encouraged to be used in several applications such as; topical blends, baths, shower salt scrub, nasal inhalers, and room spritzers to benefit the cleansing process, reduce inflammation, and create an uplifting environment.

Bergamot (*Citrus aurantium ssp. bergamia*) soothes the flow of digestion, harmonizes the liver energy, and reduces nervous indigestion and loss of appetite due to emotional stress.

Chamomile, Roman (*Anthemis nobilis*) reduces indigestion, flatulence, gastritis, abdominal pain, irregular bowel movements, and ulcerative colitis.

Grapefruit (*Citrus x paradisi*) improves the lymphatic system, clears inner heat, and thereby, clears the body of toxins.

Helichrysum (*Helichrysum italicum*) reduces inflammation, stimulates and promotes tissue repair.

Lemon (*Citrus x limon*) boosts the immune system and cleanses the body, improves the functions of the digestive system, and is helpful for constipation.

Petitgrain (*Citrus aurantium*) restores mental fatigue, confusion, and anxiety. Increases liver vitality, reduces digestive issues, and insomnia.

Yarrow (*Achillea millefolium*) is an excellent digestive aid; improves digestion, elimination, and can calm gastric spasms.

Nasal Inhaler- Citrus Happiness

This blend is effective to promote emotional uplifting.
Saturate the felt wick of a nasal inhaler with these essential oils:

- **6 drops grapefruit** (*Citrus paradisi*)
- **7 drops orange** (*Citrus sinensis*)
- **5 drops mandarin** (*Citrus reticulata*)
- **2 drops spearmint** (*Mentha spicata*)

Application: Inhale as needed to calm emotions. This blend is balancing and centering. This blend can be used throughout the day and evening.

Citrus Cleanser Dead Sea Salt Shower Scrub
Makes approximately 1 cup/ 8oz.

- ½ cup combination of each: **fine grain Dead Sea salt and sea salt**
- Mix in **two to three tablespoons of organic unrefined safflower** (*Carthamus tinctorius)* or **sesame** *(Sesamum indicum)* oil

   Essential oil blend:

- **5 drops bergamot** (*Citrus bergamia*)
- **5 drops grapefruit** (*Citrus paradisi*)
- **4 drops lemon** (*Citrus limon*)

Apply three times a week in the shower, before you turn the water on. Massage a small amount at a time with long movements along the natural lymphatic flow, towards the heart. Dead Sea salt scrubs are excellent to slough off old skin cells, increase the circulation and lymphatic flow, and can even reduce pain and inflammation.

Before use always review the essential oils precautions.
Precaution- DO NOT apply to newly shaved areas, wounds, face, or breast tissue. These citrus essential oils also have a skin irritation precaution and are NOT recommended in the bath.

All About Clay

The use of medicinal clay in folk medicine goes back to prehistoric times. The first recorded use of medicinal clay is recorded in ancient Mesopotamia. Indigenous peoples around the world still widely use clay. The American Indians were the first to use bentonite for its adsorptive properties. According to one Indian legend, a deposit of natural clay of miraculous medicinal qualities was used by the medicine men in the Bighorn Mountains of Wyoming and Montana. They called this clay "ee-wah-kee," meaning "the mud that heals."

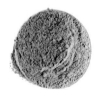

Today, a wide variety of clays are used for healing medicinal purposes.

CLAYS are a fantastic medium for hydrosols and essential oils. They can be applied as compresses, facial masks, baths, skin, and wound care. Some can even be used internally.

Clays are distinguished by their color, which is also the indicator of their structure and activity.

Green French Clay is best reserved for overactive, oily skin types. It is an active absorbent and is used primarily for drainage, where it reduces swelling, and in topical compresses for sore joints, muscles, and arthritis. Green clay is also useful for purifying and detoxing treatments.

Red Clay is also known as Rhassoul Clay. It has been used for centuries in spa applications, such as the body wraps used in Turkish bath houses.
The red color results from its high iron content. Good for deep cleansing, soothing to rough skin and is recommended for aging skin.

Pink Kaolin Clay is perfect for general, cosmetic use, offering a combination of gentleness and deep cleansing. Note: Red and Pink masks will appear to leave a light red stain behind as you first rinse them off; do not be alarmed, as it does fade almost immediately.

White Kaolin Clay is very useful for skin repair, cleansing, and toning, and it is also gentle enough for sensitive and dry skin. A very mild clay that is good as a thickening agent and does not draw oils from the skin.

Fullers Earth Clay is well known for its ability to "soak up" oils, making this one of the best clays for those who have extra oily skin types. Also, this clay is often used in facial "bleaching" masks as it holds a natural skin lightening effect that comes from its components of minerals. This is an excellent choice for those that have blemishes, light age spotting, or prone to acne.

Facial Mask

- **1 teaspoon clay**, I prefer green or Rhassoul clay
- **1 teaspoon hydrosol** (Try German chamomile *(Matricaria recutita)* or helichrysum *(Helichrysum italicum)*
- **1-2 drops essential oil**
  Essential oil recommendations: Roman chamomile *(Anthemis nobilis)*, geranium *(Pelargonium graveolens)*, lavender *(Lavandula angustifolia)*, cypress *(Cupressus sempervirens)*, or helichrysum *(Helichrysum italicum)*

Mix the ingredients in a glass bowl. Apply a thin layer of the clay mask on your face. You can also apply it to your neck and upper chest.

Since the clays are only active when wet, you can determine the intensity of activity by varying the thickness. To reduce the intensity of action, shorten the duration of treatment or decrease the thickness of the clay. To increase the intensity of action, apply a thicker layer of clay or lengthen the duration. Most masks are between 1/16 and 1/4-inch-thick, but even a fine layer of clay can be useful.

Clay Poultices are used on smaller areas for healing underlying tissues and organs, and are usually one inch thick. For normal skin allow the clay to dry.

For delicate skin, let it dry for only five to ten minutes. As the clay dries, it is pulling out toxins and impurities.

Rinse off the mask with warm water. Gently rub with a wet washcloth to remove it.

After you rinse the mask off your skin may look slightly red, which is normal and will disappear in about 30 minutes.

Finish the routine with a hydrosol spray and facial serum.

Bentonite Clay is highly absorbent and is used regularly in the cosmetics industry to add texture and volume to masks. Bentonite is hard to work into a smooth paste on its own, but is wonderful combined with Green clay. Two to four pounds added to a bath is reported to be an excellent detoxifying treatment for the body. It is highly recommended for those with exposure to paint and other chemicals.

Bentonite Clay is composed of aged volcanic ash. The name comes from the largest known deposit of Bentonite Clay located in Fort Benton, Wyoming. This is a unique clay due to its ability to produce an "electrical charge" when hydrated. It is known for its ability to absorb and remove toxins, heavy metals, impurities, and chemicals. The reason why it is so effective is its inert property, as it is not absorbed by the body. It is a substance that naturally absorbs toxins, yet does not get absorbed itself. When Bentonite clay is used internally it passes through your colon it absorbs any toxins it finds and then just passes through and is released.

Internal Use of Clay - Internal use of clay is recommended during a cleanse or one to two times a week. Mix ½ to one teaspoon of clay into four ounces of warm water. Mix well and drink. Make sure to drink plenty of pure water throughout the day.

Precautions: Not recommended if there are acute digestive issues. Not recommended for young children. Be sure to speak with your doctor while increasing your intake of clay if you are experiencing digestive issues. Don't take two hours before or after medications, and wait an hour after taking bentonite clay to eat.

Clay Bath- Bentonite clay is detoxifying and is also useful for skin issues such as eczema and psoriasis. Green clay can also be used as a substitute. Start by adding two to four cups of clay into the running bath water. Then, mix five to eight drops of essential oils into one tablespoon of jojoba (*Simmondsia chinensis*), castile soap, or Solubol, and then add this to the running bath water. Soak for 20 to 30 minutes. Rinse with clear warm water to remove the clay from your body.

Clay Bath Blends:

Mix the following ingredients together, before adding to the bath water:

Essential oil blend for detoxification and immune stimulation:

- **1 tablespoon jojoba** (*Simmondsia chinensis*), castile soap, or Solubol
- **4 drops- tea tree** (*Melaleuca alternifolia*)
- **2 drops- helichrysum** (*Helichrysum italicum*)
- **2 drops- cedarwood** (*Cedrus deodara*)

Essential oil blend for detoxification and immune stimulation:

- **1 tablespoon jojoba** (*Simmondsia chinensis*), castile soap, or Solubol
- **3 drops Roman chamomile** (*Anthemis nobilis*)
- **3 drops palmarosa** (*Cymbopogon martinii*)
- **3 drops yarrow** (*Achillea millefolium*)

These blends can also be added directly to one to two cups of bath salts or clay for additional cleansing and rejuvenation.

Spring Holistic Therapies

Spring is the perfect time for cleansing and rejuvenating the internal organs. **Chi Nei Tsang and Mayan Abdominal Therapy** are very beneficial modalities to enhance digestion, circulation, lymphatic flow, reduce stagnation and congestion. Working on the abdomen will increase your overall health and wellbeing.

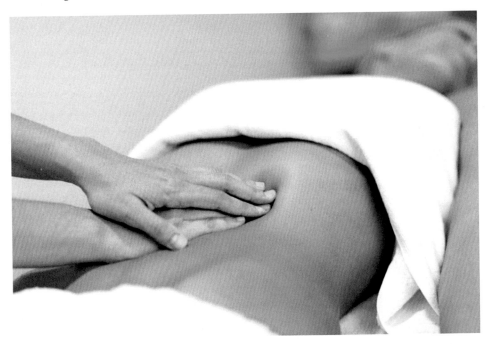

Shiatsu- focuses on stimulating specific meridian points by use of pressure techniques on acupoints often done using thumb or palms. This technique also incorporates massage kneading and effleurage. Treatments can reduce the following; headaches, PMS, digestive disorders, fatigue, insomnia, fibromyalgia, stress, anxiety, and musculoskeletal pain, including low back, neck, and joint pain.

Spring Quote

"The beautiful spring came; and when Nature resumes her loveliness, the human soul is apt to revive also."
Harriet Ann Jacobs

Chapter

Summer

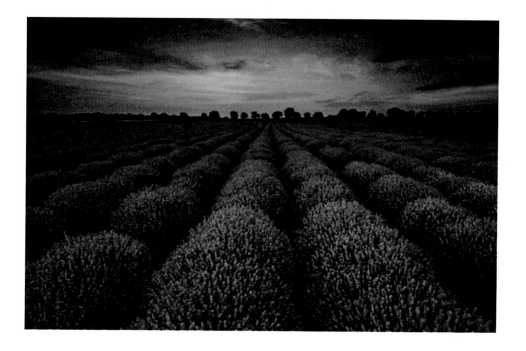

Summertime is the warmest time of year with the fastest growth. This season corresponds to the direction of the south, the warmest and brightest direction, and noontime when the sun is the highest in the sky and the light is the most brilliant.

It symbolizes the peak of energy, the time of flourishing and when we are most active and spend more time outside. The life phase of summertime correlates to the time when we shine most brightly, when we are at the top of our game, full of energy, and filled with knowledge and skill.

During summer, this expansive warmth encourages us to give and receive love, connect and relate to the world like a flower opening to full bloom.

However, if internal heat becomes excessive, one might experience issues like; excessive sweating, burning inflammation of the joints, chronic infections, hot flashes, dryness of the lungs, and inflamed throat. Excess heat can also dry out the stool and cause constipation. Emotionally, this can often be expressed by excessive rush, impatience, arrogance, anxiety, mood swings, and restlessness.

Summer Herbs

Summer is the perfect time to incorporate cooling and refreshing herbs.

These herbs can be used in tea, decoction, infusion, flower essence, or tincture form.

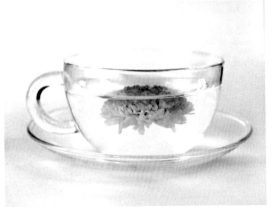

Chrysanthemum
(Chrysanthemum morrifolium)

This flower has a long and rich history in herbal medicine. It was first cultivated as an herb around the fifteenth century BC. In the west, it was first officially described by the famous botanist Karl Linnaeus, in 1753.

It is recognized for its cleansing and cooling nature, helping to assist the body rid toxic heat from the liver and clear congestion in the upper body.

Precaution: Not advised for use by those with a sensitivity to ragweed.

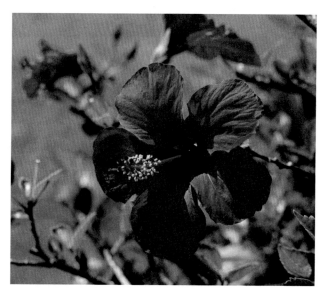

Hibiscus (*Hibiscus sabdariffa*)

This beautiful flower is widely grown throughout the world, and is used to a great extent in refreshing teas in North and South America.

Hibiscus is cooling, assists to maintain healthy body temperature, supports circulation, and encourages fluid balance.

Precaution: Hibiscus is often grown with peanut plants.
Be aware of the source of the growing area for those with a severe peanut allergy.

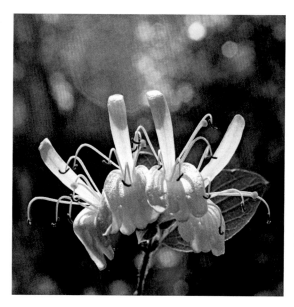

Honeysuckle
(*Lonicera periclymenum*)

This plant is sometimes referred to as "woodbine." The flower, seed, and leaves are used as medicine for urinary disorders, headache, reducing inflammation of the skin, and other heat issues. It can be used to promote sweating and as a laxative.

Honeysuckle is considered one of the 50 fundamental herbs in Chinese herbology and is often combined with chrysanthemum flowers in tea.

Summertime Sun Tea

Summer is the only time I consume a moderate amount of iced beverages. I find refreshing aromatic sun teas very delightful. You can use the herbs profiled in the previous pages or include them in a base of green tea.

Why green tea?

What is green tea's most significant benefit? "It's all about the catechin content," says Beth Reardon, RD, a Boston nutritionist. Catechins are antioxidants that fight and may even prevent cell damage. Green tea is not processed as much as other teas before it is poured in your cup, so it's rich in catechins.

What else is green tea good for?

- Improves blood flow.
- Lowers cholesterol.
- Keeps the blood sugar balanced.
- Protects brain cells from dying and restores damaged brain cells.
- The antioxidant and anti-inflammatory activities can reduce signs of aging.

Enjoy a couple of my favorite sun tea blends:

Jasmine Pearls Green Tea with Lavender Flowers and Hydrosol

In a one gallon (glass container) of **purified water**:

Add:

3 tablespoons jasmine (*Jasminum grandiflorum*) **green tea pearls**

1/2 cup of dried lavender (*Lavandula angustifolia*) **flowers**

Place the container out in the sun for one to two hours. Then, strain and refrigerate.

Once chilled, add a few cubes of ice into an eight ounce glass and add one teaspoon of **rose geranium** (*Pelargonium graveolens*) or **rose** (*Rosa damascena*) **hydrosol.**

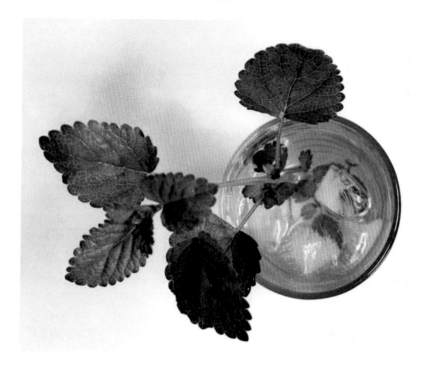

Green Tea with Peppermint and Spearmint Hydrosol

In one gallon (glass container) of purified water:

Add:

3 tablespoons organic green tea

1 cup of fresh peppermint *(Mentha piperita)*

Place the container out in the sun for one to two hours. Then, strain out the tea leaves and refrigerate. It is an option to keep the peppermint in the jar for extra flavor.

Once chilled, add a few cubes of ice into a glass and add one teaspoon of **spearmint** *(Mentha spicata)* **hydrosol**.

Summer Flower Essences

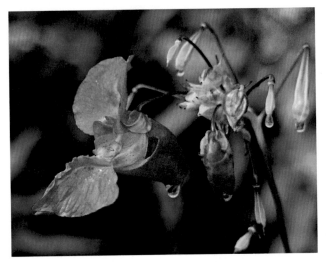

Impatiens
(Impatiens glandulifera)

Just as the name implies, this flower essence reduces impatience.

Encourages Positive Qualities:
Reduces frustration, irritability and hastiness.
This flower essence calms agitated thoughts and feelings.
Encourages relaxation with others.
"Accepting Gentle Flow"

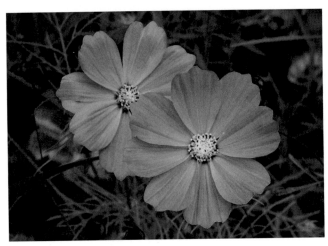

Cosmos
(Cosmos bipinnatus)

For those who feel unfocused, disorganized, and overwhelmed by too many thoughts or ideas.

Encourages Positive Qualities:
Integration and expression of ideas with clarity. This flower essence removes blockages between the heart essence and intellectual mind.
"Integrated communication."

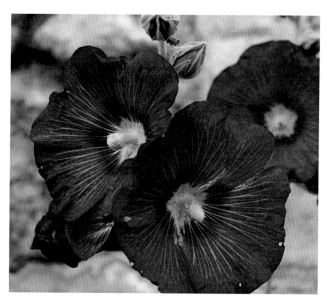

Red Hollyhock
(Alcea rosea)

For people suffering from depression, loss of faith and hope, Red Hollyhock helps them to enhance their awareness of being fully present with joy and optimism, in whatever situation they are dealing with.

This flower essence assists us in connecting with life enthusiastically and in aligning with the present moment.

Encourages Positive Qualities:
Lightening of Spirit
Joy, Optimism, and Enthusiasm
"Joyful Heart Radiance"

Summer Hydrosols

Summertime is the perfect time of year to increase your use of hydrosols. Used by themselves, or in combination, with other aromatherapy applications such as, facial spritzers and toners.

Catnip *(Nepeta cataria)*

Reduces heat and fever, used as a calming sedative for anxiety, digestive, and respiratory complaints, and to reduce insomnia. Effective in natural insect repellant sprays to avert mosquitoes, fleas, and ticks.
NOTE: Due to the high level of nepetalactone, this can be stimulating to cats.

Cucumber *(Cucumis sativus)*

Refreshing and cooling in facial toner, spritzer, or body spray. Cucumbers are well known for their soothing, healing, and anti-inflammatory effects. Used for promoting healthy skin, as well as addressing skin issues and infections; eczema, psoriasis, soothing sunburn, and reducing fine lines and wrinkles.

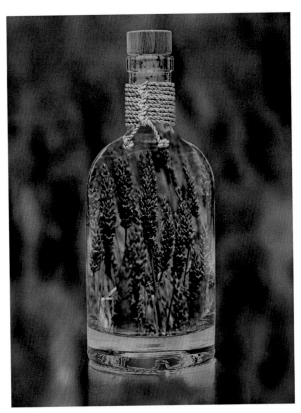

Lavender *(Lavandula angustifolia)* Of course, lavender is included in the summer hydrosols!

Wonderful sedative, reduces insomnia, and powerful anti-inflammatory.

It is a calming hydrosol that is also useful as a skin healer for cuts, wounds, sunburns, insect bites, and infections.

 Lavender hydrosol is a fantastic addition to your first aid kit.

Neroli *(Citrus aurantium)* This beautiful flower is excellent for its calming and soothing properties and to reduce anxiety. Neroli essential oil is costly, and the hydrosol makes an effective substitution for body sprays as the hydrosol does have a strong aroma. It has a soft floral and citrus aroma very similar to the essential oil. This hydrosol is useful for both skin and hair, and its astringent nature is beneficial to use in skin care products for oily skin types.

Rosemary *(Rosmarinus officinalis ct. verbenone)* hydrosol is a gentle tonic for all skin types when used in facial toners and spritzers. It assists in easing congestion, puffiness, and swelling. Used in hair care products it has a pronounced positive effect on the health of the hair and scalp, and it promotes hair growth.

Precautions: This chemotype of rosemary hydrosol is safer during pregnancy and for children. Please check additional precautions before using the essential oil. Rosemary is an adrenal stimulant and should not be used after 6pm at night to encourage a restful night's sleep.

Summer Carriers

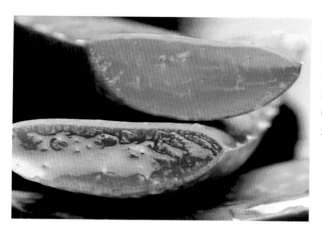

Aloe vera gel (*Aloe barbadensis*) is useful as a primary response for first aid on wounds, cuts, sunburns, and heat rashes.

Jojoba (*Simmondsia chinensis*) is actually a plant wax that has a very long shelf life. It is used as a dispersing agent in liquid blends, herbal infusions, skin care, and other aromatherapy applications.

Witch hazel extract (*Hamamelis virginiana*) apply to minor cuts and scrapes to stop bleeding. This is also useful for facial products, inflamed skin, cleaning wounds, and bug bites. The recommended witch hazel extract, which contains a lower amount of isopropyl alcohol, is available from several suppliers.

Arnica oil (*Arnica montana*) reduces inflammation and muscle fatigue, bruises, and sprains. **Precaution:** Do not apply to any open wounds or cuts.

Enjoy one of my favorite summer blends used as a refreshing facial spray:

In a 2oz. amber glass bottle with a spray top add:

- **1 tablespoon jojoba** (*Simmondsia chinensis*)
- **10 drops lavender** (*Lavandula angustifolia*)
- **8 drops palmarosa** (*Cymbopogon martinii*)
- **6 drops rose** (*Rosa damascena*)

  Then add:
- **1 oz. lavender** (*Lavandula angustifolia*) **hydrosol**
- **½ oz. witch hazel extract** (*Hamamelis virginiana*)
- **½ oz. purified water**

Refrigerate and use anytime you need a refreshing and hydrating facial spritzer.

Summer Essential Oils

Summer is my favorite season to use essential oils, absolutes and CO2s sourced from flowers.

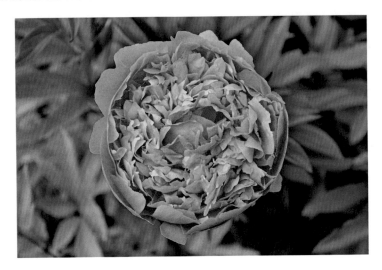

Rose *(Rosa damascena)* - Clears heat and inflammation, reduces anxiety and calms the heart. The essential oil is used for all skin types to reduce dry, sensitive skin, and inflammation. A wonderful addition to facial toner for all skin types, and is also used in body spritzers, anti-anxiety spray, deodorant, and room freshener.

Neroli *(Citrus aurantium var. amara)* - When we are overburdened or oppressed by the past and weighed down by overattachments, neroli essential oil can help us to break free. It can be used for states of agitation and worry, or when the mind is distracted and overwhelmed by thoughts. Balances both emotional and physical challenges.

Known for its uplifting scent, it is also very beneficial for the body and skin whenever you need an analgesic, antiseptic, antispasmodic, cicatrisant, or immune stimulant.

Palmarosa *(Cymbopogon martinii)* - Replenishing, cooling and hydrating, and is beneficial for inflammatory skin conditions and skin care products.

Ylang Ylang *(Cananga odorata)* – Clears heat, relaxes the mind, and calms the nerves. Assists in the release of anger and sadness and helps reconnect an individual with the child self. This oil reduces anxiety and insomnia.

The essential oils mentioned may all be diffused, put into a nasal inhaler for use three to six times per day, placed in an aroma patch, or diluted into carrier oil to be applied to the body or bath to achieve their benefits.

Summer is a time of outdoor activity and traveling. Use these easy tips to keep your immune system strong during your summer journeys:

- Wash your hands often.
- Keep your stress level as low as possible.
- Drink plenty of water.
- Get plenty of rest.
- Eat minimal refined sugar and other refined foods.

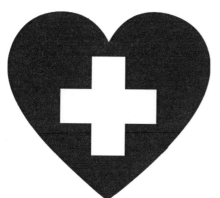

We all want to enjoy the beauty and warmth of the sun during the brightest days of summer. You can put together a first aid kit including some herbal medicinals useful for outings, taking care of insect bites, bruises, bumps, cuts, wounds, and unsettled emotions.

Summer First Aid Kit

When you put together your first aid kit, you will want to include a selection of flower essences, tinctures, hydrosols, carrier oils, essential oils, and aromatherapy blends.

Here are some suggestions to get you started.

First Aid Kit Flower Essences

- **Impatiens** *(Impatiens glandulifera)* reduces impatience, frustration, and irritability.
- **St. John's Wort** *(Hypericum perforatum)* has impressive restorative powers, providing protection and strength when a person is overwhelmed or feeling physically challenged. Also, useful for a wide variety of sleep disturbances, such as insomnia.
- **Bach rescue remedy** is a combination of five flower essences: rock rose *(Cistus ladanifer)* to alleviate terror and panic, impatiens *(Impatiens glandulifera)* to reduce irritation and impatience, clematis *(Clematis vitalba)* to combat inattentiveness, Star of Bethlehem *(Ornithogalum umbellatum)* to ease shock, and cherry plum *(Prunus cerasifera)* to calm irrational thoughts. There is also a kids rescue remedy available.

First Aid Kit Tinctures

- **Ashwagandha root** *(Withania somnifera)* reduces anxiety and stress, improves brain function, and provides hormonal support.
- **Astragalus root** *(Astragalus propinquus)* wonderful stimulant for the immune system. General tonic and effective at fighting bacteria and viruses.
- **Echinacea** *(Echinacea purpurea)* is used as first stage immune support. This herb reduces many symptoms of colds, flu, and infections.

First Aid Kit Hydrosols

- **Lavender** *(Lavandula angustifolia)* calming hydrosol, useful for cuts, wounds, sunburns, insect bites, and infections.
- **Catnip** *(Nepeta cataria)* reduces heat and fever, used as a calming spray sedative for anxiety, and to reduce insomnia. Effective in natural insect repellant spray to avert mosquitoes, fleas, and ticks.
- **Peppermint** *(Mentha piperita)* is used for mental fatigue, refreshing to the spirit and stimulating mental agility and improving concentration. It is cooling for the skin and relieves irritation, inflammation and itchiness. It is refreshing added to ice tea (½ tablespoon per 8 oz.), add to other drinks, or use as a cooling facial spritzer.
  Precautions: Not recommended for children under five. Peppermint hydrosol is an adrenal stimulant and should not be ingested four to six hours before sleep.

Keep hydrosols refrigerated whenever possible.

First Aid Kit Carriers

- **Aloe vera gel** *(Aloe barbadensis)* is cooling, soothes sunburn, rashes, cuts, and wounds.
- **Jojoba** *(Simmondsia chinensis)* is good to have on hand as a base carrier oil to mix up essential oil blends.
- **Witch hazel extract** *(Hamamelis virginiana)* is cooling, soothes sunburn, rashes, bites, cuts, and wounds.

First Aid Kit Essential Oils

- **Helichrysum** *(Helichrysum italicum)* is a most potent anti-inflammatory. Useful for healing of cuts and wounds, reducing swelling and inflammation, and promoting tissue repair.
- **Rose** *(Rosa damascena)* clears heat and inflammation, reduces anxiety and calms the heart. Useful to reduce anxiety, impatience, dry and sensitive skin, and inflammation.
- **Manuka** *(Leptospermum scoparium)* keeps infections at bay, including colds, flu, and fever. Used for muscle inflammation, cuts, wounds, and other skin infections. In my experience, Manuka is more potent and faster acting than Tea Tree *(Melaleuca alternifolia)*.

I am only highlighting three essential oils for a first aid kit; however, there are so many others that are conducive to first aid applications. You might also consider coriander *(Coriandrum sativum)*, Roman chamomile *(Anthemis nobilis)*, frankincense *(Boswellia carterii)*, lavender *(Lavandula angustifolia)*, neroli *(Citrus aurantium)*, and palmarosa *(Cymbopogon martinii)*.

First Aid Kit Aromatherapy Blends

Soothing After Sun Gel
Makes 2oz.

Combine the following ingredients into a 2oz. (60ml.) BPA-free plastic bottle with a flip top:

- **10 mls jojoba** *(Simmondsia chinensis)*
- **8 drops rose** *(Rosa damascena)*
- **8 drops lavender** *(Lavandula angustifolia)*
- **8 drops helichrysum** *(Helichrysum italicum)*

Shake well and then add the additional ingredients:

- **40 mls aloe vera gel** *(Aloe barbadensis)*
- **10 mls witch hazel extract** *(Hamamelis virginiana)*

Apply the soothing after sun gel after being in the sun for an extended period of time.

Note: only one percent dilution of essential oils (six drops total) for children and during pregnancy.

Essential oils are a very effective way to keep bugs at bay. The blend below is quite useful to repel mosquitoes, flies, and ticks.

Bug Repellent Blend
Makes 4oz.

In an 4-oz. amber glass bottle mix together:

- **1 tablespoon of jojoba** *(Simmondsia chinensis)*

Then, add in the following essential oils and shake well:

- **8 drops catnip** *(Nepeta cataria)*
- **6 drops lemongrass** *(Cymbopogon citratus)*
- **6 drops lemon eucalyptus** *(Eucalyptus citriodora)*
- **6 drops cedarwood** *(Cedrus atlantica)*
- **4 drops rosemary** *(Rosmarinus officinalis)*
- **5 drops peppermint** *(Mentha x piperita)*

Then add:

- **1 oz. aloe vera gel**

To the remainder of the bottle, add purified water or a choice of hydrosol.

- **catnip** *(Nepeta cataria)*, **lemongrass** *(Cymbopogon citratus)*, **or peppermint** *(Mentha x piperita)* **hydrosol** adds a beautiful aroma to this blend.

Decant into one to two-ounce bottles. I especially recommend using spray top bottles for ease of convenience. Label, and spray away!

For a thicker gel application you can omit the water or hydrosol.

Shake well before use. Apply as needed on the arms, legs or other exposed areas.

Precautions: This bug repellent blend is not recommended during pregnancy, for children under ten years of age, and those taking anti-cancer medications.

Compassionate Heart Blend

In a 10ml glass roller bottle mix together:

- **9.5 mls jojoba** *(Simmondsia chinensis)*
- **5 drops rose** *(Rosa damascena)*
- **5 drops neroli** *(Citrus aurantium var. amara)*
- **5 drops ylang ylang** *(Cananga odorata)*

Shake well. Apply, as needed, on the upper chest, and abdomen to reduce anxiety, and stress. This blend of essential oils can also be used in a nasal inhaler or aroma patch.

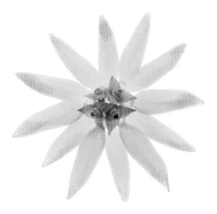

Topical Pain Relief Blend

Makes 1 oz.

Combine the following ingredients into a BPA-free plastic bottle with a flip top:

- **1 oz. arnica infused oil** *(Arnica montana)*
- **5 drops helichrysum** *(Helichrysum italicum)*
- **4 drops manuka** *(Leptospermum scoparium)*
- **3 drops lavender** *(Lavandula angustifolia)*

Apply as needed to inflamed muscles and joints, or other painful areas. **Precautions:** DO NOT apply on wounds or cuts. Not for use in the bath. Not for use with children under five years old.

Summer Holistic Therapies

Summer is a good time for light touch and energy healing modalities.

Craniosacral - improves function of the autonomic nervous system, enabling the body to respond more effectively to stress and tension. This modality can reduce or eliminate a range of imbalances including; chronic pain, central nervous system disorders, head and neck pain, temporal mandibular joint (TMJ) pain, fibromyalgia, chronic fatigue, seizure disorders, hormonal imbalances, and chronic sinus issues.

Watsu (Water Shiatsu)- used for deep relaxation, rehabilitation, and profound physical release of tension. Sessions take place in a warm therapeutic pool and is a healing modality currently practiced in hospitals, clinics, and spas.

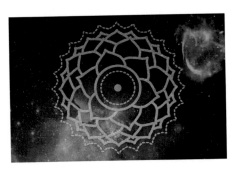

Energy work such as Medical Qigong, Reiki, and Resonance Alchemy.

These energy healing modalities encourage the body's natural tendency to return to balance and equilibrium. They improve physical and emotional health, as well as increasing higher levels of energy and stamina.

Self-Administered:

Qigong - promotes flexibility, balance, and good body awareness. It relaxes and strengthens the nervous system, decreases inflammation and stimulates the energy flow of the meridians.

Tapping - useful to reduce emotional stress and rebalancing.

Summer Quote

"The sun shines not on us but in us. The rivers flow not past, but through us. Thrilling, tingling, vibrating every fiber and cell of the substance of our bodies, making them glide and sing.
The trees wave and the flowers bloom in our bodies as well as our souls, and every bird song, wind song, and tremendous storm song of the rocks in the heart of the mountains is our song, our very own, and sings our love."
John Muir

Conclusion

It is my wish and intention, in sharing the information in this book, that you enjoy radiant health and freedom from physical and emotional sufferings.

I remember vividly as a child, around age eight, sitting on my bedroom floor playing with some toys when I experienced a lucid inner conversation, "If I am going to have to work all my life I want to spend my time on something that is meaningful." I have thought about that dynamic memory many times throughout my life. That realization led me to healing work and traveling around the world learning different healing methods. It is a blessing to be able to share this appreciation and incredible healing beauty of nature with others.

Around age twenty-seven, I recorded a few notes about my journey, thus far, and thought that someday it might be a book about my healing adventures. In my sixtieth year, I realize that I have finally acquired the knowledge and the experience to speak about natural healing from a depth of understanding; through my exploration of integrating the amazing healing powers of nature and holistic therapies into everyday life. I will continue to learn and grow as a student of the earth and healing spirit.

May you use these tools provided to develop a profound connection with nature's healing and a deeper relationship with yourself. May you know radiant health, unconditional love, and joyous experiences of life's extraordinary journey. ~

The mountains are calling, and I must go.
John Muir

References by Chapter

Chapter 1

- Book Cover and Chapter title picture; original designs created by Mark Talbot/Xplore Design; copyright owned by Shanti Dechen. https://www.xplore.design/
- Body, Mind, Soul Picture; purchased from Shutterstock; https://www.shutterstock.com/image-photo/holistic-health-concept-zen-stones-deep-1008807274?src=bhBlQPLd_bP1Qe2hhKC9cg-1-4; Retrieved September 15, 2018.
- (1) Sherry, Jane; Blog Article; SusunWeed.com; http://www.susunweed.com/herbal_ezine/May09/goddess.htm; Retrieved June 23, 2018.
- Sunflower Picture; free for commercial use; CCO Creative Commons; found on Pixabay; https://pixabay.com/en/sunflower-flower-petals-bloom-3614728; Retrieved August 20, 2018.
- (2) BBC Documentary: How Plants Communicate & Think; https://www.youtube.com/watch?v=Q-4w5xYLwiU; Retrieved May 12, 2016.
- (3) Communicative & Integrated Biology Article; http://www.ncbi.nlm.nih.gov/pmc/articles/PMC2649305/; Retrieved May 13, 2016.
- (4) Mycorrhizal Fungi http://www.mycorrhizae.com; Retrieved May 14, 2016.
- (5) Vanier, LJ; Article quoting Dr. Olivia Bader-Lee: Scientists Find Plants Are Intelligent and Communicate Telepathically; http://itsallabouti.info/scientists-find-plants-are-intelligent-and-communicate-telepathically/#7eo53zq7kPEKU3L1.99; Retrieved May 15, 2016.
- Nature Connection Picture; purchased from Shutterstock; https://www.shutterstock.com/image-photo/agriculture-growing-plants-plant-seedling-hand-362501594?src=75vRF62qnQlkRbNiL0SM4w-1-10; Retrieved October 5, 2018.
- (6) Forrester, Michael; Scientists find Plants Communicate Telepathically https://upliftconnect.com/plants-communicate/; Retrieved May 13, 2016.

Additional Resources

- Mitsch, Jacques Documentary: In the Mind of Plants https://www.youtube.com/watch?v=h33TKImM-kk; Retrieved October 3, 2018.
- PBS Documentary: What do Plants Talk About? https://www.youtube.com/watch?v=CrrSAc-vjG4 ; Retrieved October 3, 2018.

Chapter 2

- Chapter title picture; free for commercial use; CCO Creative Commons; found on Pixabay; https://pixabay.com/en/heart-love-romance-valentine-700141/; Retrieved September 26, 2018.
- Gratitude picture; purchased from Shutterstock; https://www.shutterstock.com/image-photo/gratitude-attitude-female-hand-outstretched-palm-223186420?src; Retrieved September 26, 2018.
- Colorful Heart picture; free for commercial use; CCO Creative Commons; found on Pixabay; https://pixabay.com/en/colorful-prismatic-chromatic-1237242/; Retrieved September 20, 2018.

Additional Resources

- Article: 6 Steps to Set Good Boundaries; https://www.mindbodygreen.com/0-13176/6-steps-to-set-good-boundaries.html; Retrieved June 28, 2018.
- Article: 7 Tips to Create Healthy Boundaries with Others; https://www.psychologytoday.com/us/blog/in-flux/201511/7-tips-create-healthy-boundaries-others; Retrieved June 28, 2018.
- Chopra, Deepak; 5 Steps to Setting Powerful Intentions;https://chopra.com/articles/5-steps-to-setting-powerful-intentions; Retrieved June 26, 2018.

Chapter 3- Using Medicinal Plants

- Chapter picture Medicinal Plants; purchased from Dreamstime; ID 77187322 © Julia FaranchukDreamstime.com; Retrieved September 26, 2018.
- Borage *(Borago officinalis)* picture; purchased from Shutterstock; https://www.shutterstock.com/image-photo/borage-flower-356593193?src=_au8wxyEOt_u0NcFg9J0OA-1-11; Retrieved September 28, 2018.
- Tincture and herbs picture; purchased from Shutterstock; https://www.shutterstock.com/image-photo/bottles-tincture-potion-dry-healthy-herbs-447367420; Retrieved September 4, 2018.
- Evening primrose *(Oenothera biennis)* picture; free for commercial use; CCO Creative Commons; found on Pixabay; https://pixabay.com/en/evening-primrose-plants-flowers-1458681/; Retrieved September 24, 2018.
- (1) Lyth, Geoff; What are Absolutes?; https://www.quinessence.com/absolutes; Retrieved May 11, 2018.
- Aromatherapy Mandala picture; purchased on Dreamstime; ID 55231174 © Montserrat SantanderDreamstime.com; Retrieved September 28, 2018.
- Aroma Patch picture; Used with written permission from Jodi Baglien; http://www.jodibaglien.com/about-patches/; Retrieved August 31, 2018.
- Bath Applications picture; free for commercial use; CCO Creative Commons; found on Pixabay; https://pixabay.com/en/essential-oils-aromatherapy-spa-oil-1433694; Retrieved September 22, 2018.

Chapter 4- Seasonal Wellness

- Chapter title picture; original design created by Mark Talbot/Xplore Design; copyright owned by Shanti Dechen. https://www.xplore.design/
- Earth picture; purchased from Shutterstock; https://www.shutterstock.com/image-vector/green-earth-concept-leavesvector-illustration-453384865; Retrieved September 3, 2018.
- Feet Grounded picture; purchased from Shutterstock; https://www.shutterstock.com/image-photo/young-girls-bare-feet-feeling-softness-105868442; Retrieved September 17, 2018.
- Forest bathing; http://www.natureandforesttherapy.org/about.html; Retrieved August 13, 2018.
- (1) Sonnenburg, Justin PhD. and Sonnenburg, Erica PhD.; Book Review; The Good Gut: Taking Control of Your Weight, Your Mood and Your Long-Term Health; https://www.scientificamerican.com/article/gut-feelings-the-second-brain-in-our-gastrointestinal-systems-excerpt/; Retrieved July 15, 2018.
- (2) Nasrallah, Henry A. MD.; Psychoneurogastroenterology: The abdominal brain, the microbiome, and psychiatry; http://www.mdedge.com/currentpsychiatry/article/99085/somaticdisorders/psychoneurogastroenterology-abdominal-brain; Retrieved July 15, 2018.
- (3) Gershon, Michael D.; The Enteric Nervous System: A Second Brain; https://pdfs.semanticscholar.org/070b/273d202704a18c7974186eb6a5e4e5110a54.pdf; Retrieved July 15, 2018.
- Abdomen picture; purchased from Shutterstock; https://www.shutterstock.com/image-photo/perfect-beautiful-body-young-girl-isolatedon-72063691; Retrieved September 3, 2018.
- Spices picture; free for commercial use; CCO Creative Commons; found on Pixabay; https://pixabay.com/en/spices-jar-cooking-rustic-pepper-2548653; Retrieved September 17, 2018.
- Cardamom (Elettaria cardamomum) picture; purchased from Shutterstock; https://www.shutterstock.com/image-photo/green-cardamom-pods-wooden-spoon-360070946?src=library; Retrieved September 12, 2018.
- Tierra, Michael, L.Ac., O.M.D.; The Way of Herbs, p. 74; Pocket Books; 1998.
- Coriander/Cilantro (Coriandrum sativum) picture; taken August 1, 2018; owned by Shanti Dechen.
- Turmeric (Curcuma longa) picture; purchased from Shutterstock; https://www.shutterstock.com/image-photo/composition-bowl-turmeric-powder-on-wooden-762961246?irgwc=; Retrieved September 29, 2018.
- (4) Block, Edward F.; Food Therapy for the Traditional Chinese Medicine (TCM) Diagnosis of Dampness; https://medcraveonline.com/IJCAM/IJCAM-02-00050.pdf; Retrieved December 8, 2016.
- Red Clover (Trifolium pretense) picture; free for commercial use; CCO Creative Commons; found on Pixabay; https://pixabay.com/en/klee-blossom-bloom-bloom-purple-2346760/; Retrieved September 8, 2017:
- Mullein (Verbascum thapsus) blossom picture; free for commercial use; CCO Creative Commons; found on Pixabay; https://pixabay.com/en/blossom-bloom-yellow-summer-53248/; Retrieved September 22, 2018.

- Frangipani *(Plumeria alba)* lowers picture; free for commercial use; CCO Creative Commons; found on Pixabay; https://pixabay.com/en/blossom-bloom-flower-frangipani-335327/; Retrieved September 27, 2018.
- Perfume bottles picture; free for commercial use; CCO Creative Commons; found on Pixabay; https://pixabay.com/en/still-life-roses-perfume-1460067/; Retrieved September 25, 2018.
- Bottoms of feet picture; Kidney 1 picture; purchased from Shutterstock; https://www.shutterstock.com/download/confirm/156880376?size=huge_jpg; Retrieved September 29, 2018.
- Sunrise picture; free for commercial use; CCO Creative Commons; found on Pixabay; https://pixabay.com/en/sunrise-space-outer-space-globe-1756274; Retrieved September 29, 2018.

Chapter 5- Autumn

- Chapter picture; free for commercial use; CCO Creative Commons; found on Pixabay; https://pixabay.com/en/maple-maple-leaves-emerge-2135514/; Retrieved September 28, 2018.
- Dandelion *(Taraxacum officinale)* picture; purchased from Shutterstock; https://www.shutterstock.com/image-photo/dandelion-sunset-freedom-wish-401624755?src=tmIUd6N3VkNvpOc0vE8wRg-1-8; Retrieved September 30, 2018.
- Moore, Michael; *Medicinal Plants of the Mountain West*; p. 183; Museum of New Mexico Press; revised edition; 2003.
- Echinacea *(Echinacea purpurea)* picture; free for commercial use; CCO Creative Commons; found on Pixabay;https://pixabay.com/en/echinacea-flower-plant-nature-2887013/; Retrieved September 25, 2018.
- (1) Tierra, Michael, L.Ac., O.M.D.; *The Way of Herbs: Fully Updated with the Latest Developments in Herbal Science*; pg. 132, 133; New York, NY; Pocket Books; revised edition 1998.
- Elderberry *(Sambucus nigra)* picture; free for commercial use; CCO Creative Commons; found on Pixabay; https://pixabay.com/en/elder-holler-elderberry-tree-3599629/; Retrieved September 25, 2018.
- German chamomile *(Matricaria recutita)* picture; free for commercial use; CCO Creative Commons; found on Pixabay; https://pixabay.com/en/chamomile-chamomile-blossoms-829220/; Retrieved September 25, 2018.
- Arnica *(Arnica montana)* picture; purchased from Shutterstock; https://www.shutterstock.com/image-photo/closeup-photo-yellow-arnica-80072617; Retrieved September 30, 2018.
- Calendula *(Calendula officinalis)* picture; free for commercial use; CCO Creative Commons; found on Pixabay; https://pixabay.com/en/marigold-calendula-officinalis-2666877; Retrieved September 25, 2018.
- Rosehip *(Rosa canina)* picture; free for commercial use; CCO Creative Commons; found on Pixabay; https://pixabay.com/en/rosehip-red-berries-nature-autumn-1166531/; Retrieved September 20, 2018.

- Calendula (*Calendula officinalis*) Infusion picture; purchased from Shutterstock; https://www.shutterstock.com/image-photo/marigold-extract-small-bottle-medicinal-herbs-705040375; Retrieved September 6, 2018.
- St. John's Wort (*Hypericum perforatum*) picture; free for commercial use CCO Creative Commons; found on Pixabay; https://pixabay.com/en/blossom-bloom-st-john-s-wort-374510/; Retrieved September 28, 2018.
- Creeping Bellflower (*Campanula rapunculoides*) picture; free for commercial use; CCO Creative Commons; found on Pixabay; https://pixabay.com/en/bellflower-flower-bell-bluebells-354229/;Retrieved September 29, 2018.
- Myrrh (*Commiphora myrrha*) picture; free for commercial use; CCO Creative Commons; found on Pixabay https://pixabay.com/en/myrrh-medicinal-plant-2736724/; Retrieved September 25, 2018.
- Autumn Heart Leaf picture; free for commercial use; CCO Creative Commons; found on Pixabay; https://pixabay.com/en/heart-sweetheart-leaf-autumn-maple-1776746/; Retrieved September 29, 2018.
- (2) Deng, Cynthia; Yale Scientific Article: Aromatherapy: Exploring Olfaction; http://www.yalescientific.org/2011/11/aromatherapy-exploring-olfaction/; Retrieved December 8, 2016.
- (3) XN, LV. et.al.; Aromatherapy and the Central Nerve System (CNS): Therapeutic Mechanism and its Associated Genes; PubMed Article; https://www.ncbi.nlm.nih.gov/pubmed/23531112; Retrieved December 8, 2016.
- Cedar picture; purchased from Shutterstock; https://www.shutterstock.com/image-vector/green-fluffy-cedar-branch-two-cones 533579242?src=D52NAQDnJbfwA7blwbvTaA-1-8; Retrieved October 1, 2018.
- Dead Sea Salt Scrub picture; purchased from Dreamstime; ID 126704724 © Milenie | Dreamstime.com https://www.dreamstime.com/natural-ingredients-homemade-body-sea-salt-scrub-olive-oil-white-towel-beauty-concept-skincare-organic-aroma-spa-therapy-image126704724; Retrieved September 30, 2018.
- Healing Salve picture; free for commercial use; CCO Creative Commons; found on Pixabay; https://pixabay.com/en/bees-wax-lip-balm-1951036/; Retrieved September 29, 2018.
- Acupuncture picture; free for commercial use; CCO Creative Commons; found on Pixabay; https://pixabay.com/en/acupuncture-asian-medicine-needles-2277444/; Retrieved September 27, 2018.

Chapter 6- Winter

- Chapter picture; purchased from Shutterstock; https://www.shutterstock.com/image-photo/background-snowcovered-fir-branches 224911645?src=QQykdDGU46oDF5rXKOewwg-1-31; Retrieved September 3, 2018.
- Ginger (*Zingiber officinale*) picture; purchased from Dreamstime; ID 97018962 © Margo555 | Dreamstime.com; Retrieved September 30, 2018.

- Sunflower *(Helianthus annuus)* picture; free for commercial use; CCO Creative Commons; found on Pixabay; https://pixabay.com/en/sunflower-yellow-summer-blossom-1627179/; Retrieved September 8, 2018.
- Rose Geranium *(Pelargonium graveolens var. roseum)* picture; free for commercial use; CCO Creative Commons; found on Pixabay; https://pixabay.com/en/flower-pelargonium-geranium-bloom-1085998/; Retrieved September 8, 2018.
- Aromatherapy Bath Blends picture; purchased from Shutterstock; https://www.shutterstock.com/image-photo/orchid-essential-oil-mixed-various-beauty-435329308; Retrieved September 30, 2018.
- Carrier Oils picture; purchased from Shutterstock; https://www.shutterstock.com/image-photo/bottle-yellow-cosmetic-oil-big-splash-452875306; Retrieved September 4, 2018.
- Meadowfoam *(Limnanthes alba)* picture; free for commercial use; CCO Creative Commons; found on Pixabay; https://pixabay.com/en/limnanthes-douglasii-2038361/; Retrieved September 29, 2018.
- Body Butter picture; free for commercial use; CCO Creative Commons; found on Pixabay; https://pixabay.com/en/flower-rose-cream-petal-skin-care-3141777/; Retrieved September 7, 2018.
- Hot Stone Massage picture; purchased from Shutterstock; https://www.shutterstock.com/image-photo/massage-hot-basalt-stones-beautiful-deep-399976321?src=6UoeKNpeGkP2Q-P0ZNfkBQ-1-0; Retrieved September 19, 2018.

Chapter 7- Spring

- Chapter picture; free for commercial use; CCO Creative Commons; found on Pixabay; https://pixabay.com/en/spring-background-flower-yellow-316535/; Retrieved September 30, 2018.
- Spring cleaning picture; free for commercial use; CCO Creative Commons; found on Pixabay; https://pixabay.com/en/clean-spring-putz-blade-broom-1346685/; Retrieved September 20, 2018.
- Lemons picture; free for commercial use; CCO Creative Commons; found on Pixabay; https://pixabay.com/en/lemons-citrus-fruit-blossom-3334763/; Retrieved September 26, 2018.
- (1) Haas, Elson M., M.D.; *The Detox Diet*; p. 31; Berkeley, CA; Celestial Arts Publishing; 1996.
- (2) Sage Press PDF File; Technical Data Report for Chanca Piedra; http://www.rain-tree.com/chanca-techreport.pdf; Retrieved July 12, 2016.
- Milk Thistle *(Silybum marianum)* picture; free for commercial use; CCO Creative Commons; found on Pixabay; https://pixabay.com/en/flowers-thistle-milk-thistle-purple-31452/; Retrieved September 28, 2018.
- Celandine *(Chelidonium majus)* picture; free for commercial use; CCO Creative Commons; found on Pixabay; https://pixabay.com/en/greater-celandine-blossom-bloom-116273/; Retrieved September 28, 2018.

- Pink Yarrow (*Achillea millefolium var. rosea*) picture; taken August 12, 2018; owned by Shanti Dechen.
- Ledum groenlandicum picture; free for commercial use; CCO Creative Commons; found on Pixabay; https://pixabay.com/en/flower-nature-plant-spring-3271945/; Retrieved September 28, 2018.
- (3) Catty, Suzanne; *Hydrosols: The Next Aromatherapy*; p. 105-106; Rochester, VT; Healing Arts Press, 2001.
- Different types of cosmetic clay picture; purchased from Shutterstock; https://www.shutterstock.com/image-photo/various-kinds-cosmetic-clay-on-white-1048446196; Retrieved September 20, 2018.
- Appropedia; Medicinal Clay; http://www.appropedia.org/Medicinal_clay; Retrieved July 20, 2017.
- Abdominal massage; picture; purchased from Shutterstock; https://www.shutterstock.com/image-photo/hands-massaging-female-abdomentherapist-applying-pressure-716471500; Retrieved September 26, 2018.

Additional Resources

- Willmont, Dennis; *Aromatherapy with Chinese Medicine*; Marshfield, MA; Willmountain Press; 2003.
- Kaminski, Patricia, and Katz, Richard; *Flower Essence Repertory: A Comprehensive Guide to North American and English Flower Essences for Emotional and Spiritual Well-Being*; Nevada City, CA; The Flower Essence Society; Earth-Spirit Inc.; 1996.

Chapter 8- Summer

- Chapter title picture; purchased from Shutterstock; https://www.shutterstock.com/image-photo/stunning-landscape-lavender-field-sunset-192460559; Retrieved September 3, 2018.
- Chrysanthemum (*Chrysanthemum morrifolium*) picture; free for commercial use; CCO Creative Commons; found on Pixabay; https://pixabay.com/en/cup-tea-chrysanthemum-tea-681680/; Retrieved September 19, 2018.
- Hibiscus (*Hibiscus sabdariffa*) picture; free for commercial use; CCO Creative Commons; found on Pixabay; https://pixabay.com/en/hibiscus-red-blossom-bloom-flower-1554734/; Retrieved September 19, 2018.
- Honeysuckle (*Lonicera periclymenum*) picture; free for commercial use; CCO Creative Commons; found on Pixabay; https://pixabay.com/en/flower-honeysuckle-perfume-2613671/; Retrieved September 19, 2018.
- Green Tea picture; free for commercial use; CCO Creative Commons; found on Pixabay; https://pixabay.com/en/ice-tea-melissa-officinalis-840631/; Retrieved September 28, 2018.
- Impatiens (*Impatiens glandulifera*) picture; free for commercial use; CCO Creative Commons; found on Pixabay; https://pixabay.com/en/balsam-flower-blossom-bloom-pink-408530/; Retrieved September 27, 2018.

- Cosmos (*Cosmos bipinnatus*) picture; free for commercial use; CCO Creative Commons; found on Pixabay; https://pixabay.com/en/cosmos-bipinnatus-garden-cosmos-20628/; Retrieved September 27, 2018.
- Hollyhock (*Alcea rosea*) picture; free for commercial use; CCO Creative Commons; found on Pixabay; https://pixabay.com/en/mallow-hollyhock-flower-stock-rose-15338; Retrieved September 27, 2018.
- Lavender (*Lavandula angustifolia*) bottle picture; free for commercial use; CCO Creative Commons; found on Pixabay; https://pixabay.com/en/lavender-bottle-plant-spring-1490788/; Retrieved September 27, 2018.
- Aloe Vera Plant (*Aloe barbadensis*) picture; free for commercial use; CCO Creative Commons; found on Pixabay; https://pixabay.com/en/aloe-aloe-vera-life-bless-you-2163120/; Retrieved September 25, 2018.
- Rose (*Rosa damascena*) picture; free for commercial use; CCO Creative Commons; found on Pixabay; https://pixabay.com/en/damascena-damask-flowers-garden-111435/; Retrieved September 24, 2018.
- First Aid Heart picture; free for commercial use; CCO Creative Commons; found on Pixabay; https://pixabay.com/en/first-aid-medical-medicine-doctor-2789562/; Retrieved September 27, 2018.
- Ylang Ylang (*Cananga odorata*) picture; purchased from Shutterstock; https://www.shutterstock.com/image-photo/flower-arrangement-climbing-ylangylang-ilangilang-manorangini1114434116?src=dZOSWj9h_31p1QwV0t3XpA-2-37; Retrieved September 30, 2018.
- Mandala picture; free for commercial use; CCO Creative Commons; found on Pixabay; https://pixabay.com/en/chakra-crown-chakra-spiritual-2972452/; Retrieved September 27, 2018.

Index

mental fatigue, 58, 108, 126
meridians, 20
Mességué, Maurice, 105
microcosm, view of, 8
migraines, 4, 20, 86
milk thistle (*Silybum marianum*), 104
mimosa *(Acacia mirensi)*, 61
mimosa *(Albizia julibrissin)*, 38
mind, and emotions, 22
mindfulness moment, 25
mind-gut connection, 53
mood issues, 55, 76, 116
Moore, Jessica, 64
motherwort (*Leonurus cardiac*), 71
Muir, John, 52, 81, 130, 131
mullein (*Verbascum thapsus*), 60
muscle fatigue, 123
musculoskeletal pain, 114
mycorrhizal fungi, 11
myofascial release, 18
myrrh (*Commiphora myrrha*), 37, 72
myrtle, green (*Myrtus communis*), 107

N
nasal inhalers, 40, 75, 76–77, 108
Nasrallah, Henry A., 54
National Institute of Occupational Safety and Health, 99
Native American perspective, 49
nature
    body as hologram of, 20
    connection with, 5
    incorporation of into everyday language, 6
    time in as supportive and nourishing, 17
    as uplifting, energizing, and healing, 12
    walking in as beneficial for connecting deeper with Earth element, 51
naturopathy, 4, 45
nausea, 42, 86
neroli (*Citrus aurantium var. amara*), 5, 38, 61, 80, 89, 93, 122, 124, 127, 129
neuromuscular, 18
neurons, similarities of with plant cells, 10
nitrosamines, 99
O
oakmoss (*Evernia prunastri*), 61
odor messages, 76
oil face wash application, 94
olfaction/olfactory system, 5, 75, 76
olive (*Olea europaea*), 32, 70, 86, 91
orange (*Citrus sinensis*), 101, 108
oregano (*Origanum vulgare*), 89
osha (*Ligusticum porteri*), 67
osmanthus (*Osmanthus fragrans*), 61
overworking, 17

P

Q

R

Tierra, Michael, 57
tinctures, 17, 28, 31, 32, 67, 71, 85, 86, 104, 116, 125, 126
topical applications, of essential oils, 43
Topical Pain Relief Blend, 90, 129
Total Person Facilitation, 49
traumatic events, and journeys of self-discovery, 49
triethanolamine (TEA), 99
tuberose (*Polianthes tuberosa*), 37, 38, 61, 62
turmeric (*Curcuma longa*), 56, 59
U
unconditional love, as powerful healer, 3
Upledger, John, 20
urinary issues, 84, 105, 117

V
vanilla (*Vanilla planifolia*), 37, 61, 62
vegetable capsules, 32
vetiver (*Vetiveria zizanoides*), 41, 51, 61, 88, 93
violet leaf (*Viola odorata*), 38, 61
vitamin supplements, as supportive and nourishing, 17
Volkmann, Dieter, 9

W
water, element of as connected to winter, 84
Watsu (water shiatsu), 130
The Way of Herbs (Tierra), 57
well-being, individual as ultimately responsible for, 3
wellness, three great treasures to cultivate for, 29
wheat germ (*Triticum vulgare*), 80, 95
white kaolin clay, 110
winter
    as all about baths, 87–89
    body care tips for, 84
    carrier oils for, 91–94
    described, 84
    fear as emotion associated with, 85
    flower essence, 86
    herbals, 85–86
    holistic therapies, 96
    hydrosol, 87
witch hazel extract (*Hamamelis virginiana*), 123, 126, 127
woodbine, 117
wounds, 59, 69, 72, 79, 80, 87, 107, 109, 122, 123, 125, 126, 127

Y
Yale Scientific, 76
yarrow (*Acheilia millefolium*), 6, 68, 107, 108, 113
yellow dock (*Rumex crispus*), 104
ylang ylang (*Cananga odorata*), 88, 124, 129
    yoga, 4, 20, 51

ABOUT THE AUTHOR

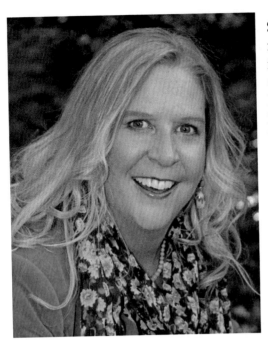

Shanti's extensive training includes many modalities of healing including;
Certified Clinical Aromatherapy Practitioner and Teacher, Herbology, Plant Medicine, Massage Therapy (including Deep Tissue) and other healing modalities well as Chi Nei Tsang: Visceral Rejuvenation, Bodymind Clearing, Lymphatic Drainage, Acupressure, Craniosacral Therapy, Asian Healing Arts, Applied Kinesiology, Polarity, Medical Qigong, Nutrition, Reflexology, Energy Medicine, Stress Management and Meditation.

Shanti has worked in clinical settings and studied in a variety of healing modalities for the last thirty-eight years in the US, Canada, Germany, Thailand, and the Caribbean. This lifelong passion of natural healing led her to establish and direct Aroma Apothecary Healing Arts Academy since 2002.

Shanti is a professional member in good standing with the NAHA (National Association of Holistic Aromatherapy), AIA (Alliance of International Aromatherapists), Senior Instructor of Chi Nei Tsang through the Universal Healing Tao and is a professional member of good standing with NCBTMB (National Certification for Therapeutic Massage and Bodywork) Practitioner and Approved CE Provider, and NAHA Regional Director of Colorado.

To learn more about the true essence of aromatherapy, visit LearnAroma.com

Made in the USA
Lexington, KY
11 October 2018